641.5   Keane, M.
Kea   The what to eat if you
            have cancer cookbook.

DEMCO

The WHAT to EAT if YOU HAVE CANCER COOKBOOK

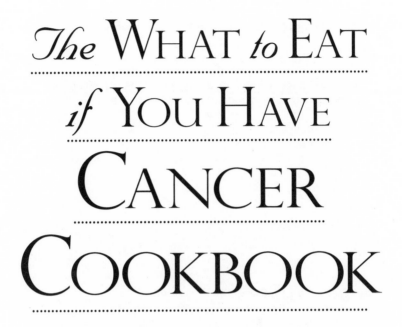

*Over 100 Easy-to-Prepare Recipes
for Patients and Their Families
and Caregivers*

**MAUREEN KEANE, M.S., AND
DANIELLA CHACE, M.S.**

CB
CONTEMPORARY BOOKS

6 4 1 . 5

Library of Congress Cataloging-in-Publication Data

Keane, Maureen.
    The what to eat if you have cancer cookbook: over 100
easy-to-prepare recipes for patients and their families and
caregivers / Maureen Keane and Daniella Chace.
      p.   cm.
    Includes index.
    ISBN 0-8092-3129-8
    1. Cancer—Diet therapy—Recipes.   I. Chace, Daniella.
II. Title.
RC271.D52K428   1997
641.5'631—dc20   96-33483
                                                CIP

Cover design by Kim Bartko
Cover painting by Charlotte Segal: *Passionata*; 1994 (oil on
canvas; 44 inches × 66 inches). Copyright © Charlotte Segal.

Charlotte Segal is an instructor at the International Academy
of Design Chicago and a 21-year cancer survivor. Segal's
paintings and prints are part of numerous corporate and private
collections. "Making art is my way to live beyond the years God
has granted me. I feel I have survived through sheer will. Further,
I view being able to create art as a gift to be treasured."

Her work is included in Healing Legacies, an arts registry that
contains work by women and men who have experienced breast
cancer. Created in 1993, the registry now represents more than
100 artists and contains more than 500 pieces of visual and
written work. For more information about Healing Legacies,
contact the Breast Cancer Action Group, PO Box 5605,
Burlington, VT 05402. Artists wishing a prospectus should
send a SASE.

Published by Contemporary Books
An imprint of NTC/Contemporary Publishing Company
4255 West Touhy Avenue, Lincolnwood, Illinois 60646-1975
Manufactured in the United States of America
International Standard Book Number: 0-8092-3129-8
15   14   13   12   11   10   9   8   7   6   5   4   3   2   1

*This book is dedicated to Daniella's mother,
Linda Chace, who inspired her nutrition studies.*

Contents

Acknowledgments

This book would not be possible without the talents of our two head recipe development chefs, who took the nutritional protocols for cancer patients and turned them into delicious recipes. We thank Linda Chace and Tonja Hill for their hard work and talents.

We would like to thank Dr. Joe Pizzorno, Dr. Deb Brammer, Dr. Jay Littel, Dr. Allan Gaby, and Dr. John Lung for their professional advice; Darren Hill for contributing his valuable experience and feedback; our recipe development assistants: Carmen Hill, Sabrina Lamb, Sally Nicholls, Susan Messina, Kristen O'Reilly, and Juanita Young; Far East culinary consultant Susan Keller (no relation); Six-Toe McFadden—feline sleep aid; and Ben Hattrup for his editorial assistance.

Introduction

Get ready for the fun part of cancer therapy!

This cookbook is designed to be a companion to *What to Eat if You Have Cancer: A Guide to Adding Nutritional Therapy to Your Treatment Plan*. It translates the dietary guidelines detailed in that book into recipes so delicious the whole family will enjoy them.

What to Eat if You Have Cancer explains how the body defends itself against cancer and the powerful link food plays in this battle. It recommends specific foods that show promise in slowing cancer growth. You probably remember your mother nagging you to eat your vegetables. Today most medical and health professionals support her advice. Fruits and vegetables are wonderful sources of energy, vitamins, minerals, and phytochemicals, which are substances found in whole foods. Some phytochemicals can block the initiation and promotion of cancer; others prevent cancer's spread or hinder the nourishment of cancer cells. Phytochemicals work synergistically to fight cancer on all these levels. Understanding which foods to eat can help you mount your best defense against this disease. For thorough discussions of tumor-inhibiting fatty acids and cancer-fighting cruciferous vegetables and soy foods, refer to *What to Eat if You Have Cancer*.

Each chapter in this cookbook highlights a specific food group and its cancer-fighting components. Because cancer therapy can cause a variety of gastrointestinal problems, it also includes chapters on soothing nutritious meals in a glass and raw fresh juices.

Enjoy this variety of nutritious and tasty recipes and know that you are enhancing the effectiveness of your cancer treatment with every bite.

To your health and recovery,
Daniella Chace and Maureen Keane

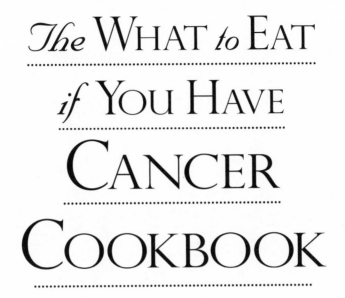

The WHAT to EAT if YOU HAVE CANCER COOKBOOK

I

Vegetables and Fruits

~~~~~

Fruits and vegetables are excellent sources of vitamins, minerals, and phytochemicals. Citrus fruits supply vitamin C and bioflavonoids; leafy green vegetables provide carotenoids and minerals; orange-colored vegetables such as carrots provide vitamin A; starchy root vegetables such as potatoes and sweet potatoes provide complex carbohydrates; and sea vegetables provide ultratrace and trace minerals. The following are some of the many benefits of these foods.

- Vitamin C acts synergistically with vitamin E as a cytotoxic agent, which can change chemically transformed cells back to normal. It is also necessary for the collagen production needed for a strong cancer-resistant connective tissue structure.

- The carotenoids, a group of yellow to red pigments, inhibit cancer initiation, increase the body's monocytes (a type of white blood cell), and reduce damage from radiation.

- Vitamin A produced from beta-carotene affects the later stages of cancer promotion and proliferation; inhibits DNA manufacture and protein synthesis of cancer cells; and increases messenger RNA levels that can alter gene expression.

- The flavonoids, another large and varied class of pigments, function primarily as antioxidants.

- Organosulfur compounds found in Allium species (garlic, onions, shallots, and leeks) prevent cancer formation and aid in breaking down and ridding the body of cancer-causing chemicals.
- Glutathione, an antioxidant, protects cells from oxygen damage.

Preparation of Fruits and Vegetables

Always wash *all* fruits and vegetables thoroughly in a cleaning solution before you eat them. Whenever possible, buy organic produce. Peel any nonorganic or waxed produce before eating to minimize your exposure to pesticides. We strongly recommend that all cooked vegetables be steamed. This prevents the loss of water-soluble vitamins to the cooking liquid. An alternative is to use a small amount of cooking water and incorporate it into the recipe.

Leafy greens and other delicate vegetables can be cooked in a food steamer. Plastic food steamers are reasonably priced and convenient to use. A good substitute is a metal steamer basket in a saucepan with a tight-fitting lid.

Root vegetables and hearty dishes such as soups and stews are best prepared in a pressure cooker. This cooking method is not only fast but also seals in nutrients and prevents potentially nauseating food odors from building up in the kitchen.

Wakame Soup

....

1 medium winter squash, cut in half and seeded

6 cups water

1 teaspoon extra-virgin olive oil

1 cup diced yellow onion

¼ cup dried wakame (see Sea vegetables/seaweed
in Glossary)

¼ cup reduced-salt tamari *or* soy sauce

1. Place the squash and ¾ cup of the water in a covered
   saucepan and steam over medium heat until tender,
   about 15 minutes. Drain and set aside.
2. Heat the olive oil in a large stockpot. Add the onion and
   sauté over medium-low heat for 2 minutes.
3. Add the remaining water to the stockpot with onion.
   Bring to a boil and reduce heat to medium.
4. Scoop the squash out of its skin with a large spoon and
   cut into 1-inch pieces. Add squash, wakame, and tamari
   to the stockpot and cook over medium-low heat for an
   additional 10 minutes.
5. If you have any leftover cooked grains, beans, or fresh
   vegetables, add them to the mixture.
6. Serve with cooked fish, beans, salad, Rocket in a Pocket
   (see Index), or whole grains.

Makes 10 servings

Winter Warm-Up Soup

....

1 medium sweet winter squash, cut in half and seeded
1 teaspoon extra-virgin olive oil
1 medium yellow onion, chopped, *or* 1 leek, sliced thin
4 garlic cloves, halved
1 small jalapeño, sliced and seeded
½ cup cubed firm tofu
2 tablespoons miso dissolved in 2 cups water
¼ cup chopped cilantro
¼ lime

1. Place squash in a covered saucepan with ½ inch of water and steam over low heat until soft, about 15 minutes. Set aside.
2. Heat the olive oil in a large pan. Add the onion, garlic, jalapeño, and tofu and sauté over medium-low heat until onion is translucent.
3. After squash has cooled to the touch, scoop the flesh into a blender.
4. Add miso broth to the blender and process on medium to high speed until smooth.
5. Add pureed squash to the pan with garlic, jalapeño, onion, and tofu. Cook until the mixture is heated through.
6. Pour soup into serving bowls and garnish with cilantro and a squeeze of lime juice.

~ *Makes 2 servings*

.

Miso

Miso is a paste made from fermented soybeans and sea salt mixed with grains such as rice or barley. It is a versatile flavoring, which comes in many varieties ranging from mild and sweet to very hot and spicy. (See Glossary.)

Eggless Caesar Salad

....

3 tablespoons flaxseed oil
¼ cup fresh squeezed lemon juice
3 garlic cloves, minced or crushed
¼ teaspoon sea salt
1 head romaine lettuce, torn into bite-size pieces
¼ cup freshly shredded Parmesan cheese

1. In a large salad bowl combine flaxseed oil, lemon juice, garlic, and salt. Mix well.
2. Add lettuce to the bowl and toss with dressing and shredded Parmesan.

⸛ Makes 4 servings

Danger: Eggs

Raw eggs should not be eaten due to their bacterial content; especially by those with compromised immune systems. This Caesar dressing is as delicious and robust in flavor as the original raw egg–containing recipe and features a substantial amount of the natural antibiotic garlic.

Cucumber Salad

....

4 large cucumbers, peeled and sliced thin
½ cup thinly sliced red onion
1 clove garlic, minced
¼ cup rice vinegar
1 tablespoon flaxseed oil
1 teaspoon chopped fresh dill

1. In a medium serving bowl, combine all ingredients.
2. Chill the salad for 2 hours in the refrigerator before serving.

Makes 8 servings

Hijiki, Carrot, and Ginger Salad

1½ cups dried hijiki, rinsed
1 tablespoon extra-virgin olive oil
3 carrots, scraped and shredded
½ teaspoon freshly grated ginger
1 tablespoon reduced-sodium tamari
1 tablespoon mirin (see Glossary)
2 teaspoons sesame seeds

1. Cover the hijiki with water and soak for 10 minutes to reconstitute. Drain.
2. Heat the olive oil in a saucepan. Add the hijiki and sauté over medium-low heat for 5 minutes.
3. Add carrots and ginger to the pan and cook for an additional 5 minutes.
4. Remove the pan from the heat. Add tamari, mirin, and sesame seeds and toss. Transfer to a serving dish.
5. Serve immediately as a hot side dish or cover and refrigerate for at least an hour and serve as a cold entree salad.

 ~ *Makes 4 servings*

Hijiki

Hijiki is a mild seaweed found in gourmet markets, health food stores, and Asian specialty shops. Seaweeds are rich in the minerals iron, calcium, potassium, and phosphorus. This Asian salad contains tangy fresh ginger, which aids digestion.

Jicama Salad

2 cups peeled and cubed jicama (see Glossary)
2 cups quartered mushrooms
1 cup coarsely chopped celery
¼ cup chopped cilantro
¼ cup chopped fresh parsley
1 medium carrot, chopped coarse
1 cup chopped tomato
¼ cup diced red bell pepper
Eggless Caesar Salad dressing (see Index)

1. Place all vegetables in a large bowl and toss with the dressing.
2. Refrigerate for 1-2 hours before serving.

～ *Makes 6 servings*

Mango Nut Salad with Poppy Seed Dressing

¼ cup slivered almonds

DRESSING

2 tablespoons flaxseed oil
¼ cup balsamic vinegar
1 tablespoon brown rice syrup
2 tablespoons poppy seeds
1 tablespoon orange juice concentrate

SALAD

1 ripe mango, cut into bite-size pieces
1 medium tomato, chopped
¼ cup chopped celery
¼ cup slivered red bell pepper
¼ cup thinly sliced red onion
1 head Bibb lettuce, torn into bite-size pieces

1. Place almond slivers into a dry frying pan and toast over medium-low heat until golden brown. Remove from heat and set aside.
2. Place all the dressing ingredients in a large salad bowl and mix well with a whisk.
3. Place salad ingredients and toasted almonds into the salad bowl and toss well. Serve immediately.

Makes 4 servings

Spinach Salad

DRESSING

4 tablespoons balsamic vinegar
2 tablespoons flaxseed oil
2 tablespoons poppy seeds
1 teaspoon dry mustard
¼ teaspoon dried barley malt syrup

SALAD

1 bunch fresh spinach, torn into bite-size pieces
1 cup thinly sliced mushrooms
3 Roma tomatoes, chopped coarse

1. In the bottom of a large salad bowl, combine the dressing ingredients and whisk together to mix well.
2. Add spinach, mushrooms, and tomatoes. Toss well to coat with dressing. Serve immediately.

Makes 4 servings

Lemon Salad Dressing

You can use this versatile dressing on salad greens, over vegetables, or as a marinade.

- 2 tablespoons flaxseed oil
- 3 tablespoons lemon juice
- 3 tablespoons tamari
- 1 tablespoon chopped fresh marjoram
- 1 tablespoon chopped fresh basil

1. Place all ingredients in a clean jar, cover, and shake.
2. Use immediately, or store it in the refrigerator for up to 1 week.

~ *Makes about ½ cup*

Asparagus with Red Peppers

1 pound asparagus stalks, trimmed and cut into thirds
1 large red bell pepper, sliced into long thin strips
3 tablespoons extra-virgin olive oil
2 tablespoons sesame seeds

1. Place asparagus and red pepper strips in a covered saucepan with 1 inch of water and steam over a low heat until tender but still crisp.
2. Toss the hot asparagus and pepper strips with olive oil and sesame seeds and serve immediately.

Makes 6 servings

Green Bean Stir-Fry

....

1 tablespoon extra-virgin olive oil

5 cloves garlic, chopped coarse

3 cups young tender organic green beans

¼ cup water

3 tablespoons low-sodium tamari

2 tablespoons oyster sauce

1 red bell pepper, sliced

1. Heat the olive oil in a large pan. Add the garlic and sauté until it begins to brown.
2. Add beans and water. Cover and steam for 5 minutes.
3. Add tamari, oyster sauce, and bell pepper. Steam for 1 additional minute and serve.

⌒ Makes 4 servings

Mashed Jerusalem Artichokes with Garlic

....

1 pound Jerusalem artichokes, peeled and cut into pieces
4 garlic cloves
3 tablespoons chopped fresh parsley
¼ cup unflavored fortified soy milk
½ tablespoon lemon juice

1. In a large pot of boiling water, boil artichokes and garlic for 25-30 minutes. Drain well.
2. Place the artichokes and garlic in a large bowl. Using a potato masher, mash the artichokes with the garlic, parsley, soy milk, and lemon juice.
3. Serve warm.

Makes 4 servings

The Allium Family

Garlic, onions, shallots, and leeks are all members of the Allium family. Their distinctive odor and flavor comes from organosulfur compounds (including diallyl sulfide, diallyl disulfide, allyl mercaptan, and alyl methyl disulfide). These agents block carcinogen activation, increase carcinogen detoxification, and block the action of tumor promoters.

Baked Rutabaga Fries

¼ teaspoon dried basil

¼ teaspoon dried rosemary

½ teaspoon paprika

1 large russet potato, peeled and sliced into ½-inch strips

1 rutabaga, peeled and sliced into ½-inch strips

1 tablespoon extra-virgin olive oil

1 drop hot pepper oil (optional)

1 tablespoon canola oil

1. Preheat oven to 350°F. Crush basil, rosemary, and paprika together in a mortar and pestle.
2. Place potato and rutabaga strips in a large bowl and toss with olive and hot pepper oils and crushed herbs.
3. Lightly oil two baking sheets with canola oil and arrange the potato and rutabaga strips in a single layer.
4. Bake strips for 15–20 minutes, turning occasionally, until lightly browned.
5. Loosen the fries with a spatula and serve on a platter with Tofu Ketchup (see Index) for dipping.

~ *Makes 2 servings*

Mashed Sweet Potatoes and Carrots

....

2 large sweet potatoes, peeled and diced
4 large carrots, peeled and diced
¼ cup barley malt syrup
¼ teaspoon sea salt

1. Place potatoes and carrots in a saucepan with 2 cups of water. Bring to a boil, reduce heat, and simmer until the vegetables are tender, about 20 minutes. Drain.
2. Mash the potatoes and carrots with a potato masher or mixer.
3. Mix syrup and salt together, pour over potatoes, and serve immediately.

Makes 4 servings

Stuffed Tomatoes

....

1 cup quinoa, rinsed (see Glossary)

1 tablespoon plus 1½ teaspoons miso dissolved in
     1½ cups water

¼ teaspoon dried thyme

½ teaspoon dried parsley

¼ cup cilantro

3 tablespoons freshly grated Parmesan cheese

¾ cup finely chopped celery

6 large firm tomatoes

1. Cook quinoa in miso broth in a saucepan until all liquid is absorbed, about 20 minutes. Remove from heat.
2. Add thyme, parsley, cilantro, Parmesan, and celery to the quinoa. Mix well and set aside.
3. Preheat oven to 350°F. Remove stems from the tomatoes and scoop out the centers. Fill each hollowed-out tomato with some of the quinoa mixture.
4. Place tomatoes in a baking dish with ¼ cup water and cover with foil. Place baking dish in oven and bake (tomatoes will steam in their own juices) for 15–20 minutes until tomatoes are cooked through.

Makes 6 servings

Sautéed Rutabagas

1 teaspoon extra-virgin olive oil
2 rutabagas, peeled and cut into long strips
1 tablespoon lemon juice
1½ teaspoons miso dissolved in ½ cup water
Salt and pepper to taste
1 cup hot cooked brown rice or other whole grain

1. Heat the olive oil in a large pan, and sauté the rutabaga strips over medium-low heat for 5 minutes.
2. Add lemon juice, miso broth, salt, and pepper and continue cooking until the vegetables are tender, about 20 minutes.
3. Serve over hot rice.

Makes 2 servings

Caramelized Vegetables over Potatoes

2 large potatoes, peeled and cubed
3 tablespoons miso dissolved in 3 cups water
2 rutabagas, peeled and diced
1 turnip, peeled and diced
2 large carrots, diced
1 medium yellow onion, chopped
1 teaspoon dried thyme
Dash of nutmeg
1 tablespoon flaxseed oil
3 tablespoons minced fresh parsley
¼ cup thinly sliced scallion

1. Place potato cubes in a saucepan with 2 cups of the miso broth and bring to a boil. Reduce heat and simmer until the potatoes are tender. Drain and reserve the liquid.
2. While potatoes are cooking, place rutabagas, turnip, carrots, and onion in another saucepan with thyme, nutmeg, and the remaining cup of miso broth. Bring to a boil and cook until all the liquid evaporates, about 10 minutes.
3. Continue to cook and stir until the vegetables are caramelized, about 10 more minutes.
4. Mash potatoes with a potato ricer or mixer and add flaxseed oil and parsley. Soften with the reserved liquid.

5. Place a mound of mashed potatoes on each of four dinner plates. Cover the potatoes with a generous ladle of the caramelized vegetables.
6. Sprinkle scallion slices over each serving.

～ *Makes 4 servings*

Pyrenees Country Stew

....

1 medium winter squash, cut in half and seeded
1 tablespoon extra-virgin olive oil
1 medium yellow onion, chopped
6 cloves garlic, minced
1 large potato, peeled and diced
2 cups shredded cabbage
½ cup split peas
1½ cups water
3 tablespoons miso
1 15-ounce can lima beans, drained

1. Place squash in a saucepan with ½ inch of water and steam for 10 minutes on low heat. Cover, remove from heat, and leave to cool.
2. Heat the olive oil in a large pan. Add the onion and garlic and sauté over medium-low heat until the onion is translucent.
3. Add potato, cabbage, split peas, water, and miso. Bring to a boil, then reduce heat and simmer for about 30 minutes.
4. When the squash is cool to the touch, cut it into bite-size pieces.
5. Add squash and lima beans to the stew and continue to cook until they are heated through.

Makes 4 servings

Pasta with Dried Fruit

....

3 tablespoons extra-virgin olive oil
4 cloves garlic, minced
¼ cup finely chopped dried papaya
¼ cup finely chopped dried cherries
¼ cup finely chopped dried apricots
2½ tablespoons balsamic vinegar
2 Roma tomatoes, diced
12 ounces pasta of choice

1. Heat olive oil in a large pan. Add garlic and sauté over medium-low heat until lightly browned.
2. Add the fruit, vinegar, and tomatoes. Cook on low heat for 20 minutes. Cover and keep warm.
3. Cook pasta as directed on the package. Drain thoroughly and toss with dried-fruit sauce.

Makes 6 servings

Fruit with Orange Sauce

SAUCE

¼ cup honey
2 tablespoons orange blossom water
⅛ teaspoon nutmeg

FRUIT

3 oranges, peeled and sectioned
2 cups sliced fresh strawberries
3 bananas, sliced
1 tablespoon chopped fresh mint

1. In a small saucepan, bring honey, orange blossom water, and nutmeg to a low boil.
2. Cook until the sauce thickens slightly, about 7 minutes. Set aside to cool.
3. In a large bowl combine fruit, mint, and cooled sauce. Toss to glaze the fruit pieces evenly and chill for 3–4 hours.

Makes 4 servings

Tasty Medicine

Glutathione is both an antioxidant and an anticarcinogen. It is present in high concentrations in oranges, cantaloupe, strawberries, peaches, avocados, asparagus, squash, cauliflower, broccoli, and tomatoes. Glutathione is destroyed by heat, so processed or cooked fruits and vegetables are not good sources.

2

....

Cruciferous Vegetables

The cruciferous family is a large group of vegetables that is so loaded with cancer-fighting agents and nutrients that it deserves separate consideration from other vegetable families. Cruciferous vegetables include leaf vegetables such as bok choy, brussels sprouts, Chinese cabbage, common head cabbage, collard greens, kale, mustard greens, and turnip greens; root vegetables such as horseradish, radish, and turnip; flower vegetables such as cauliflower and broccoli; stem vegetables such as kohlrabi; and seeds such as mustard.

Although these vegetables differ in nutritional form depending on which part of the plant is eaten, they all contain a number of anticancer compounds, including:

- Sulfur compounds (isothiocyanates and sulfuraphane), which protect cells from toxic chemicals by stimulating the production of detoxification enzymes.
- Glucosinolates (glucobrassicin and glucotropaeolin), which block and suppress cancer formation and increase carcinogen detoxification.
- Indoles, which regulate estrogen metabolism so that this hormone does not promote breast cancer.
- Vitamin C, an antioxidant that protects the watery areas of cells from the free radical damage of chemotherapy and radiation.

- Phenols (flavonoids and curcumin), which may inhibit tumor development, neutralize free radicals, and inhibit the formation of cancer-causing nitrosamines.
- Carotenoids (beta-, alpha-, and gamma-carotenes, luteine, lycopene), which retard cancer cell growth, increase cell differentiation, and neutralize free radicals.
- Glutathione (Brassica genus), an antioxidant that protects vitamin E levels in the body.
- Selenium, a trace mineral that is an important component of glutathione and represses cell proliferation.

Cooking Crucifers

The sulfur compounds in the cruciferous family are responsible for these vegetables' characteristic aroma and flavor. Heat increases the amount of sulfur compounds, so the longer they cook the more odor they produce. To preserve vitamins and reduce cooking odors that may stimulate nausea, eat these vegetables raw, blanched, or lightly steamed. A pressure cooker will help to seal in cooking odors as long as pressure is released by cooling the cooker in cold water. Juicing these vegetables produces a mild-flavored beverage that often is more appealing than the cooked vegetable.

When preparing cauliflower and broccoli, remember that the health benefits of the plant are not confined to the flowers. The stalks are nutritious as well, so don't throw them out! Just trim off the outer ⅛ inch of the stalk skin and eat the tender stalk.

Cream of Cauliflower Soup

5 tablespoons miso dissolved in 5 cups water
1 medium head cauliflower, chopped
2 stalks celery, chopped
2 cloves fresh garlic, minced
¼ cup chopped red onion
1 teaspoon curry powder
1 teaspoon dried basil
⅛ teaspoon cayenne
Salt to taste

1. Place miso broth in a large saucepan.
2. Add the cauliflower, celery, garlic, and onion and cook over medium heat for 10 minutes.
3. Stir in the curry powder, basil, cayenne, and salt and cook for 5 more minutes.
4. Place about half the vegetables and all the liquid in a blender and process until smooth and creamy.
5. Combine remaining vegetables with puree.
6. Serve hot accompanied by bread with tahini and honey.

Makes 8 servings

Cruciferous Soup

....

½ cup yellow split peas, rinsed and picked clean
4 tablespoons miso dissolved in 4 cups water
1 cup sliced carrots
1 cup chopped cauliflower
1 cup chopped broccoli
1 cup sliced red onion
1 14-ounce can stewed tomatoes
5 cloves garlic, sliced
1 tablespoon chopped fresh ginger
1 teaspoon mustard seed
1 teaspoon ground cumin
¼ teaspoon pepper

1. In a saucepan, cook the split peas in 2 cups of the miso broth for 30–40 minutes until the peas are tender.
2. Pour cooked peas and cooking broth into a blender and process until smooth and creamy. Set aside.
3. Place the remaining miso broth and the rest of the ingredients in an empty saucepan. Cook over medium-low heat for 15 minutes.
4. Pour the pea puree from the blender over cooked vegetables and stir to combine. Serve in individual bowls.

Makes 8 servings

Curried Coconut Cabbage

1 small head green cabbage, shredded
2 tablespoons miso
2 teaspoons curry powder
1 13½-ounce can low-fat coconut milk
2 teaspoons extra-virgin olive oil
1 small yellow onion, chopped
4 garlic cloves, sliced
1 red bell pepper, diced
1½ teaspoons mustard seed
Salt to taste

1. In a covered saucepan with about 1 inch of water, steam the shredded cabbage until it is well cooked, about 8 minutes. Drain well.
2. Add the miso, curry, and coconut milk and continue to simmer for an additional 2 minutes. Remove from heat and set aside.
3. Heat the oil in a frying pan. Add the onion, garlic, bell pepper, mustard seed, and salt and sauté over medium-low heat until the onion is translucent. Set aside.
4. Pour the cabbage mixture into a blender and process until creamy and smooth.
5. Combine pureed cabbage with the sautéed ingredients. Pour into soup bowls to serve.

~ *Makes 2 servings*

Coleslaw

....

2 cups shredded cabbage
1 cup grated carrot
1 8-ounce can crushed pineapple, drained
¼ cup rice vinegar
½ teaspoon caraway seeds
Salt and pepper to taste

1. In a large salad bowl combine all the ingredients and mix well.
2. Chill for at least 1 hour before serving.

∽ Makes 4 servings

Wilted Green Salad

SALAD

¼ bunch watercress, chopped coarse
¼ head bok choy, chopped coarse
¼ head kale, chopped coarse
¼ head collard greens, chopped coarse

DRESSING

¼ cup freshly squeezed lemon juice
¼ cup tamari
1 8-ounce can water chestnuts, drained

1. In a large pot, bring 1 quart of water to a boil.
2. Add watercress and cook for 1–2 minutes until the watercress turns bright green and the texture is just slightly crunchy, about 2 minutes. Drain and set aside.
3. Repeat with the rest of the greens, cooking each type separately.
4. Place dressing ingredients in a large salad bowl. Add the cooked greens and toss well.
5. Serve warm or cold.

Makes 4 servings

Cajun Brussels Sprouts

....

2 cups fresh or frozen brussels sprouts
1 tablespoon extra-virgin olive oil
½ cup chopped yellow onion
½ cup cubed firm tofu
1 14-ounce can stewed tomatoes
Pinch of thyme
Pinch of paprika
Pinch of salt
Pinch of cayenne
Pinch of black pepper

1. In a steamer or small saucepan with 1 inch of water, steam brussels sprouts for 20 minutes. Remove from the heat, drain, and set aside.
2. Heat the olive oil in a large pan. Add the onion and tofu and sauté over medium-low heat for 5 minutes.
3. Add steamed brussels sprouts to the pan and continue to sauté for another 10 minutes until the vegetables are lightly browned.
4. Stir in tomatoes and seasonings and continue to cook until tomatoes are heated through, about 2 minutes.
5. Serve over cooked whole grains, such as brown rice, quinoa, or barley, or as a side dish by itself.

Makes 4 servings

Steamed Cabbage with Apple

½ medium head cabbage, shredded
½ cup water
Pinch of salt
Pinch of pepper
Pinch of nutmeg
¼ teaspoon horseradish
½ apple, sliced

1. Place the cabbage, water, and salt in a saucepan. Cover and cook over medium-high heat for 10 minutes. Remove lid near the end of the cooking to allow the water to evaporate.
2. Add the pepper, nutmeg, horseradish, and apple and stir well.
3. Cook until the cabbage is the desired texture.

Makes 2 servings

Glazed Broccoli

....

2 cups chopped fresh broccoli
1 medium red onion, sliced thin
1 tablespoon rice vinegar
1 tablespoon brown mustard
1 tablespoon honey
1 tablespoon toasted sesame seeds

1. In a steamer or large pan with 1 inch of water, steam the broccoli and onion over medium heat until broccoli is tender. Drain and set aside.
2. In a small bowl, combine vinegar, mustard, and honey.
3. Stir the honey glaze into vegetables until they are evenly coated.
4. Serve over cooked whole grains, such as brown rice, quinoa, or barley.
5. Garnish with toasted sesame seeds.

Makes 2 servings

Cauliflower with Curry Lentil Sauce

2 cups cauliflower florets
½ cup water
¾ cup lentils, washed and picked clean
1 teaspoon lemon juice
1 teaspoon extra-virgin olive oil
1 teaspoon curry powder
¼ teaspoon turmeric
Pinch of cayenne
2 tablespoons chopped fresh parsley

1. In a steamer or small saucepan with 1 inch of water, steam the cauliflower over medium-low heat until it is tender.
2. While the cauliflower is cooking, add water and lentils to a second pan and cook over medium heat for about 15 minutes.
3. Add lemon juice, olive oil, curry, turmeric, and cayenne to cooked lentils and continue to cook, stirring, for another 5 minutes.
4. Divide the cooked cauliflower among 4 plates. Ladle the lentil sauce over cauliflower.
5. Sprinkle each serving with parsley and serve.

Makes 4 servings

Brassica Stir-Fry

¼ cup crumbled dried wakame (see Glossary)
¼ cup fresh lemon juice
8 ounces firm tofu, cubed
1 tablespoon soy sauce
1 tablespoon extra-virgin olive oil
1 cup chopped rutabaga
2 medium carrots, cut into strips
1 cup small broccoli florets
1 cup chopped cabbage
½ red bell pepper, cut into strips
½ cup chopped yellow onion
5 cloves garlic, sliced
½ teaspoon Sucanat (see Glossary)
½ cup pine nuts *or* slivered almonds

1. In a small bowl, combine wakame and lemon juice and let stand 10 minutes.
2. In a medium bowl, stir the tofu into the soy sauce and set aside.
3. Heat the olive oil in a large pan. Add rutabaga and carrot and sauté over medium heat for 3 minutes.
4. Add broccoli, cabbage, bell pepper, onion, and garlic to the pan. Sauté, stirring, for another 5 minutes.
5. Add the tofu, reconstituted wakame and lemon juice, sweetener, and nuts and sauté for 5 additional minutes.
6. Serve over a cooked whole grain, such as brown rice or kamut.

Makes 8 servings

Stir-Fry Variations

Use curly kale in place of the cabbage or cauliflower in place of the broccoli.

Soba Noodles with Wilted Kale

....

1 bunch kale, chopped
1 cup cooked soba noodles
¼ cup chopped scallion
4 tablespoons raw sesame seeds
1 tablespoon flaxseed oil
¼ cup tamari

1. In a large pot of boiling water, immerse kale until it turns bright green, about 30 seconds. Drain and place in a large bowl.
2. Add the remaining ingredients to the bowl, toss, and serve.

∼ Makes 2 servings

Soba

Soba noodles are made from whole wheat or buckwheat and should be cooked according to instructions on the package (the cooking time depends on the thickness of the noodles).

3

Grains, Nuts, and Seeds

According to the USDA's food pyramid, a healthy diet is based on grains. Each day's menu should provide 6–11 servings of grains, preferably in the form of whole grains. Unfortunately, many of us are familiar with only two grains, wheat and rice. To fully experience the health benefits whole grains have to offer, we need to eat a much wider variety. Some grains you may be familiar with are barley, buckwheat, millet, oats, rye, and wild rice. More unfamiliar grains include amaranth, kamut, spelt, quinoa, and teff.

If you have cancer, you should eat only whole grains, as refined grains lack the mineral- and vitamin-rich germ and fiber-containing bran.

Grains provide most of the basic nutrient needs of the body including:

- Protein. All grains (with the exception of corn) contain all of the essential amino acids. The body needs protein to strengthen the immune system and to rebuild cells damaged by cancer treatments.
- Fiber. Whole grains are an excellent source of both soluble and insoluble fiber. Rice and wheat are good sources of the insoluble fiber that pulls water into the colon and aids in the prevention and treatment of constipation. Oats are rich in insoluble fiber and work to normalize the gut, relieving both constipation and diarrhea. A high-fiber diet

also regulates insulin release, which keeps blood sugar levels from climbing too high and feeding cancer cells.

- Complex carbohydrates. Grains are the best source of this form of time-release energy.
- B vitamins. Grains also contain the vitamins necessary to release the energy and nutrients from foods, including thiamin, riboflavin, and niacin.
- Beta glucans. Found in oats, these substances have natural antibiotic properties.
- Vitamin E. This fat-soluble vitamin works as an antioxidant to protect the fats in cell membranes. It also reduces inflammation. Some studies have shown that it may prevent cancer cell spread. The selenium found in whole grains works together with the vitamin E to act as a powerful antioxidant.

Cooking Grains

Grains can be cooked in three ways: on the stove, in a food steamer, or in a pressure cooker. Each method has its own benefits. The stove-top method is cheapest because it requires no special equipment. The disadvantage is that you have to watch the pot to make sure that it does not burn. On the other hand, it is almost impossible to burn grains in a food steamer and the cooked product comes out fluffy, never gummy. The pressure cooker is the fastest method, cooking whole grains in less than 10 minutes.

We recommend the food steamer for delicate fast-cooking grains—such as amaranth, buckwheat, millet, quinoa, teff, and cracked grains—and the pressure cooker for longer-cooking hearty grains such as barley, brown rice, kamut, rye, oats, spelt, wheat, and wild rice.

Cooked grains can be served hot or cold with milk and fruit as a breakfast cereal, served with cooked vegetables as a dinner grain, made into a pudding for desserts, or ground into a flour for breads and other baked products.

Each type of whole grain is a unique composition of nutrients. Most of the recipes in this section can be made with a number of different grains. Experiment! If you cannot find some of the more exotic grains in your grocery or health food store, there are addresses in the back of this book for mail order.

Breakfast Grains

....

1 cup raw grains (whole oats, wheat, rye, millet, or
a blend)
¼ teaspoon salt
4 cups water

The Night Before

1. Place all the ingredients in the upper part of a double
boiler.
2. Cover and cook for 30-60 minutes depending on the
hardness of the grains.
3. Remove from heat, cover, and let stand overnight.

In the Morning

4. Reheat and serve with honey and soy milk.

⁓ Makes 4 servings

Quinoa Pudding

....

1 cup quinoa

3 cups apple juice

½ cup finely chopped dried pears, apples, *or* prunes

¼ cup raisins *or* currants

½ cup shelled pumpkin seeds

¼ teaspoon cinnamon

¼ teaspoon nutmeg

1. Place all ingredients in a saucepan and bring to a boil.
2. Reduce heat and continue cooking for 15 minutes. Add water if necessary to keep pudding from burning.
3. Place half the mixture in a blender and process until creamy. Mix with remaining cooked quinoa.
4. Chill in refrigerator for at least 2 hours.
5. Serve with soy milk or topped with a dollop of yogurt.

Makes 6 servings

Tabbouleh Salad

....

1¼ cups bulgur

4 cups water

¾ cup chopped scallion

1 cup chopped tomato

1½ cups chopped fresh mint *or* parsley

½ cup fresh lemon juice

¼ cup flaxseed oil

¼ teaspoon freshly ground pepper

1. Place bulgur in a large bowl.
2. In a medium saucepan, heat the water to the boiling point and then pour it over the bulgur. Let stand for 1 hour, or until all liquid is absorbed.
3. Add the scallion, tomato, and mint and stir to mix well.
4. Add the lemon juice, flaxseed oil, and pepper. Mix well and chill in the refrigerator until ready to serve.

Makes 6 servings

Healthy Fats

Flaxseed oil contains omega-3 polyunsaturated fatty acids, which inhibit tumor growth and stimulate the immune system's defenses against cancer growth.

Miso Rice and Broccoli

2 cups brown rice
4 tablespoons miso dissolved in 4 cups water
1 teaspoon turmeric
1 cup chopped broccoli

1. Place rice, miso broth, and turmeric in a saucepan with a tight-fitting lid and bring to a boil.
2. Reduce heat and simmer on low heat for 30 minutes (do not open the lid).
3. Add broccoli, stir, replace lid, and simmer for an additional 7 minutes.

~ *Makes 8 servings*

Yellow Rice with Miso

2 cups coconut milk

1 cup brown rice

2 tablespoons miso

1½ teaspoons turmeric

¼ teaspoon sea salt

1. Combine all ingredients in a large saucepan. Bring to a boil, then reduce heat and simmer for about 40 minutes until all the liquid is absorbed.

Makes 4 servings

Nutty Wild Rice

2 cups wild rice
3 tablespoons miso dissolved in 3 cups water
½ cup chopped almonds *or* pecans
½ cup chopped celery
1 tablespoon orange juice concentrate
1 cup chopped mushrooms

1. Cook rice in miso broth as directed on the package.
2. While the rice is cooking, toast nuts in a dry skillet over medium heat, stirring constantly, until they begin to brown. Remove from heat.
3. When the rice has finished cooking, add the nuts and the remaining ingredients and mix well. Serve warm or cold.

⁓ Makes 8 servings

Lemon Parsley Rice

....

2 cups brown rice

3 tablespoons miso dissolved in 3 cups water

¼ cup lemon juice

¼ cup Parmesan cheese

¼ cup chopped fresh parsley

1. Combine rice and miso broth and bring to a boil. Reduce heat and cover. Cook until all the liquid has been absorbed, approximately 45 minutes.
2. Add the remaining ingredients and mix well.

~ *Makes 6 servings*

Garlic and Ginger Fried Rice

2 tablespoons sesame oil
¼ teaspoon hot chile oil
3 cloves garlic, chopped
1 tablespoon finely chopped fresh ginger
1 cup firm tofu, sliced in thin strips
3 cups cooked brown rice
1 cup fresh snow peas
½ cup chopped broccoli
1 tablespoon tamari
2 tablespoons oyster sauce

1. Heat the sesame and chile oils in a large sauté pan. Add garlic and ginger and sauté over medium heat until garlic is golden brown.
2. Add tofu and continue to sauté for 1 minute.
3. Add rice, snow peas, broccoli, tamari, and oyster sauce. Cover and simmer for 2–3 minutes. Serve hot.

~ *Makes 4 servings*

Gamasio

....

4 tablespoons white sesame seeds
4 tablespoons black sesame seeds
1 teaspoon sea salt

1. In a dry frying pan over medium heat, toast sesame seeds until they begin to brown.
2. While the seeds are still hot, crush with a mortar and pestle or grind in a food processor.
3. Add salt.
4. Sprinkle gamasio over grain dishes as an alternative to using salt. It can be stored in the refrigerator for up to two days.

Makes about ½ cup

Granola Bars

½ cup honey
½ cup barley malt syrup
2 cups oats
1 cup chopped walnuts
¾ cup chopped almonds
⅓ cup flaxseeds
¼ cup sunflower seeds
¾ cup raisins
¾ cup dried cherries
½ teaspoon cardamom
¼ teaspoon cinnamon

1. Preheat the oven to 350°F.
2. In a medium saucepan combine honey and barley malt syrup and cook at a low boil for 5 minutes.
3. Remove the pan from the heat and immediately add the rest of the ingredients. Mix well.
4. Line a 9″ × 13″ pan with wax paper and pour in the mixture, making sure that it is evenly distributed across the pan.
5. Bake for 14 minutes or until golden brown.
6. Let cool for 30 minutes. Cut into squares and serve.

Makes 12 bars

Ginger Raisin Cookies

....

¾ cup applesauce

½ cup molasses

1 tablespoon soy flour

2¼ cups whole wheat flour

1 cup oats

1 cup raisins

1 teaspoon cinnamon

1 teaspoon powdered ginger

½ teaspoon ground cloves

½ teaspoon ground nutmeg

½ teaspoon salt

¼ teaspoon baking soda

¼ teaspoon aluminum-free baking powder

2 tablespoons canola oil

1. Preheat the oven to 350°F.
2. In a large bowl mix applesauce, molasses, and soy flour and beat until creamy.
3. Add the remaining ingredients except the canola oil and mix well.
4. Lightly oil two baking sheets with canola oil. Drop cookie dough 1 tablespoon at a time onto baking sheets.
5. Bake for 10 minutes.

⚘ *Makes 2 dozen cookies*

Power Cookies

⅓ cup soy flour

1 cup barley flour *or* whole wheat flour

1 cup rolled oats

1 teaspoon cinnamon

½ teaspoon baking soda

½ teaspoon salt

1 tablespoon vegetable oil

½ cup barley malt syrup *or* maple syrup

⅔ cup low-fat coconut milk *or* water

1 teaspoon coconut extract

2 tablespoons orange juice concentrate

½ cup chopped dried apricots *or* dried prunes

¼ cup flaked coconut

1 tablespoon canola oil

1. Preheat oven to 350°F.
2. In a large bowl, mix together flours, rolled oats, cinnamon, baking soda, and salt.
3. In another bowl, combine vegetable oil, barley malt syrup, coconut milk or water, coconut extract, and juice concentrate.
4. Add the dry mix to the wet ingredients and combine thoroughly.
5. Stir in the dried fruit and the flaked coconut.
6. Lightly oil a baking sheet with canola oil. Drop cookie dough 1 tablespoon at a time onto the baking sheet. Mash each cookie flat with a wet fork. Bake for 20 minutes.

Makes 18 cookies

4

....

Protein Foods

~~~

For many of us, protein means red meat. But when you have cancer you must learn to expand that definition to include other more healthful sources of protein. This chapter stresses recipes made with high-protein legumes and fish.

Legumes are plants that belong to the pea family. The dried edible seeds of these plants are beans, lentils, and peas. Legumes come in enough colors, sizes, shapes, and textures to suit every occasion and taste. Soybeans and foods made from them are also legumes, but because of the special properties of soy foods they will be considered in a separate chapter. Next to grains, legumes should be one of the most common foods the cancer patient eats. Nutritional components of legumes include:

- Protein, which is necessary to rebuild tissues injured during cancer treatments and to keep the immune system working at full strength.
- Insoluble fiber, which slows the release of glucose into the bloodstream, keeping sugar levels balanced so that they cannot feed the cancer tumor. Insoluble fiber is also fermented by bacteria in the colon, producing short-chain fatty acids (SCFAs). These SCFAs help prevent colon cancer.
- Protease inhibitors, which inhibit cancer formation.
- Saponins, which enhance immunity, are toxic to some cancer cells, and inhibit DNA synthesis in tumor cells.

Soaking and Cooking Times for Beans

Type of Bean	Soaking (hours)	Cooking	Pressure Cooker (soaked beans)	Pressure Cooker (unsoaked beans)
Adzuki beans	4	1 hour	15 minutes	20 minutes
Black beans	4	1½ hours	15 minutes	20 minutes
Black-eyed peas	-	45 minutes to 1 hour	-	10 minutes
Cannellini beans	4	1 to 1½ hours	15 minutes	20 minutes
Dals	-	30 minutes	-	8 minutes
Fava beans	12	3 hours	40 minutes	1 hour
Garbanzo beans	4	2 to 2½ hours	25 minutes	30 minutes
Great Northern beans	4	1 hour	20 minutes	25 minutes
Kidney beans, red	4	1 to 1½ hours	20 minutes	25 minutes
Kidney beans, white	4	1 hour	20 minutes	25 minutes
Lentils, brown	-	35 minutes	-	12 minutes
Lentils, green	-	40 minutes	-	12 minutes
Lentils, red	-	30 minutes	-	8 minutes
Lima beans	4	1 to 1½ hours	20 minutes	25 minutes

Type of Bean	Soaking (hours)	Cooking	Pressure Cooker (soaked beans)	Pressure Cooker (unsoaked beans)
Mung beans	4	45 minutes to 1 hour	-	-
Navy beans	4	2 hours	25 minutes	30 minutes
Pigeon peas	-	30 minutes	-	10 minutes
Pinto beans	4	1 to 1½ hours	20 minutes	25 minutes
Red Mexican beans	4	1 hour	20 minutes	25 minutes
Split peas	-	30 minutes	-	10 minutes
Soybeans	12	3 to 3½ hours	30 minutes	35 minutes

Preparing Beans

Beans can be purchased in several forms: fresh, frozen, canned, and dried. The most economical way to purchase beans is in bulk from a bin. The frozen varieties are more expensive but require less preparation and cooking. Canned beans are precooked; they are the easiest to use, and the most convenient.

Before you prepare dried beans, inspect them for debris and rinse them. Dried beans must be rehydrated before they can be cooked. The easiest way is to soak them overnight in salted water. A pressure cooker can be used to presoak beans quickly by adding 3 cups of salted water for each cup of dried beans. The beans are pressure-cooked for five minutes and the pressure is let it fall on its own. Whichever method you use, afterward the beans should be drained and rinsed of the salt before proceeding with the recipe. Count on dried beans doubling their volume after soaking. Split peas, black-eyed peas, and lentils do not require presoaking.

Always discard the soaking and cooking water. Some of the oligosaccharides responsible for flatulence-producing properties of beans are lost to the water. When you are ready to cook the soaked beans do not salt the cooking water. Salt at this stage will prevent water absorption and toughen the skin.

If you are going to cook dried beans, it is best to invest in a pressure cooker. Ordinary cooking methods take anywhere from 30 minutes to 1 hour. Pressure cookers cut the time substantially.

Different types of beans require different cooking times. Always read package instructions before soaking and cooking. See chart, Soaking and Cooking Times for Beans, on pages 56-57.

Bean Spread

....

2 cups cooked soybeans
1 cup vegetable juice
1 tablespoon flaxseed oil
1 cup chunky salsa
2 tablespoons chopped fresh parsley

1. In a blender or food processor fitted with a metal blade, process the soybeans with ½ cup of the vegetable juice until creamy.
2. Slowly add the remaining juice until the mixture is a uniform consistency.
3. Add flaxseed oil and salsa and blend for another 30 seconds.
4. Spread the mixture on slices of whole grain bread or serve as a dip with raw vegetables. Sprinkle parsley over the top.

Makes 4 servings

Creamy Hummus

....

1 16-ounce can garbanzo beans
2 medium lemons, juiced
1 teaspoon sea salt
½ cup water
3 tablespoons flaxseed oil
3–4 cloves garlic
½ cup tahini (ground sesame paste)
1 teaspoon chopped fresh mint

1. In a blender or food processor fitted with a metal blade, puree the garbanzo beans, lemon juice, salt, water, oil, garlic, and tahini until creamy.
2. Stir in mint and serve the hummus immediately with toasted pita wedges, raw vegetables, or crackers. It also makes a great spread on sandwiches.

~ *Makes 3 cups*

Hummus Variations

For a Southwestern flavor add a roasted bell pepper and a teaspoon of cumin to the puree and omit the mint.

To increase the calorie content of the recipe add 2 more tablespoons of flaxseed oil. Each tablespoon of oil adds 120 calories and 14 grams of healthy fat.

Baked Beans

....

1 tablespoon extra-virgin olive oil
½ medium yellow onion, chopped
3 cloves garlic, sliced
2 cups cooked beans (adzuki, kidney, or pinto)
1 tablespoon molasses
1 tablespoon tamari
1 teaspoon dry mustard
1 tablespoon canola oil

1. Preheat the oven to 350°F.
2. Heat the olive oil in a small pan. Add the onion and garlic and sauté over medium-low heat until the onion is translucent.
3. Combine the onion mixture with the beans, molasses, tamari, and mustard. Lightly oil a baking dish with canola oil. Add the bean mixture.
4. Bake for 20 minutes, or until golden brown.

Makes 4 servings

Bean Burger Mix

....

½ cup dried garbanzo beans
¼ cup dried soybeans
¼ cup dried lentils
¼ cup shelled sunflower seeds
¼ cup peanuts
¼ cup rolled oats
¼ cup cornmeal
¼ cup wheat germ
2 tablespoons soy flour
2 tablespoons nutritional yeast
1 tablespoon dried parsley
1 teaspoon baking soda
2 teaspoons sea salt
1⅔ cups hot water
3–5 teaspoons tamari *or* soy sauce
¾ cup extra-virgin olive oil

1. In a blender or food processor fitted with a metal blade, process beans, seeds, nuts, and oats to the consistency of a coarse flour. Process ½ cup at a time for best results.
2. Combine with the remaining dry ingredients. (This dried mixture can be stored in a closed container in the refrigerator for up to 2 weeks.)
3. Now you're ready to form the patties. For each two patties, add ⅓ cup of hot water to 1 cup of dry mix and let stand for 15 minutes. For a saltier flavor, add a teaspoon of tamari as the mixture soaks.
4. Wet hands and form two thin patties.

5. Heat 2 tablespoons of the oil in a medium sauté pan. Add the patties and fry each side for about 4 minutes, until browned.
6. Add 1 tablespoon of water to the pan, cover, and continue to cook for 2 minutes.
7. Repeat, cooking two patties at a time, to make the desired number of servings.
8. Serve on whole wheat hamburger buns with Tofu Ketchup (see Index), onions, and lettuce.

Makes 10 patties

Falafel in a Pocket

FALAFEL

2 cups cooked garbanzo beans
½ cup water
½ cup whole wheat flour
2 cloves garlic, minced
1 tablespoon tahini
1 tablespoon flaxseed oil
¼ cup chopped Italian parsley
¼ teaspoon cumin
¼ teaspoon dried basil
¼ teaspoon cayenne
¼ cup extra-virgin olive oil

SPICY GARLIC SAUCE

2 medium tomatoes, chopped
2 scallions, chopped
2 cloves garlic, chopped
½ cup chopped Italian parsley
¼ cup nonfat yogurt
1 tablespoon flaxseed oil
½ teaspoon tamari
½ teaspoon cumin

6 pita pockets, slit

1. In a large bowl, mash beans with a fork or potato masher. Slowly pour in water, flour, garlic, tahini, flaxseed oil, and seasonings.
2. Form mixture into small balls, about 1 inch wide.
3. Heat olive oil in a frying pan. Add the falafel balls and sauté over medium heat until they are cooked through. Drain on paper towels while you make the sauce.
4. In a medium bowl, combine all the sauce ingredients. Mix well. (Store any unused sauce in refrigerator for up to 2 days.)
5. Place the falafel balls inside pita pockets. Drizzle the sauce over the falafel or serve with the sauce on the side.

⌇ Makes 6 servings

Rocket in a Pocket

....

2 cups cooked garbanzo beans
½ teaspoon dried basil
3 cloves garlic, crushed
2 tablespoons lime juice
½ teaspoon paprika
½ medium yellow onion, chopped fine
½ cup finely chopped celery
½ cup chopped fresh parsley
3 tablespoons flaxseed oil
3 cups finely chopped fresh rocket (arugula)
1 large tomato, chopped
6 pita pockets

1. Mash the beans with a potato masher and add basil, garlic, lime juice, and paprika.
2. Stir in onion, celery, parsley, and flaxseed oil and mix well.
3. Combine rocket and tomato into the mixture.
4. Slit pita pockets and fill with the mashed mixture and serve immediately.

~ *Makes 6 servings*

Arugula

Arugula (pronounced ah-ROO-guh-lah) is also known as rocket. Arugula originated in the Mediterranean and western Asia. This tender, mustard-flavored green is slightly bitter and aids in digestion.

Lentil Herb Loaf

1 tablespoon extra-virgin olive oil
½ medium yellow onion, chopped
4 cloves garlic, sliced
2 cups cooked lentils
2 teaspoons miso dissolved in ½ cup water
½ cup wheat germ
½ cup chopped walnuts
1 tablespoon balsamic vinegar
1 tablespoon tamari
1 teaspoon thyme
1 tablespoon canola oil

1. Preheat the oven to 350°F.
2. Heat olive oil in a small pan. Add the onion and garlic and sauté over medium heat until onion is translucent.
3. Mix all ingredients together. Lightly oil a loaf pan with canola oil. Place the lentil mixture in the pan and mold it into a loaf. Bake, covered, for 30 minutes.
4. Uncover and bake for an additional 10 minutes.

Makes 8 servings

Black Bean and Spinach Lasagna

TOMATO SAUCE

2 tablespoons extra-virgin olive oil
1 medium yellow onion, chopped fine
3 cloves garlic, chopped fine
1 28-ounce can crushed organic tomatoes
1 8-ounce can tomato paste
½ teaspoon sea salt
4 sprigs fresh rosemary
1 teaspoon fennel seed
1 teaspoon sweet dried basil

TOFU SAUCE

2 14-ounce packages firm tofu
½ medium yellow onion, chopped fine
2 cloves garlic, chopped fine
2 tablespoons tamari

THE REST

18 dried or fresh lasagna noodles, cooked according to
   package directions
1 bunch whole spinach leaves, stems pinched off
1 15-ounce can black beans, rinsed and drained
½ cup freshly grated Parmesan cheese

1. Preheat the oven to 350°F.

2. To make the tomato sauce, heat olive oil in a heavy saucepan. Add the onion and sauté over medium-low heat until it becomes translucent. Add the remaining sauce ingredients, cover, and simmer for 20 minutes.

3. While the tomato sauce is cooking, place all the tofu sauce ingredients in a food processor and blend thoroughly. Pour tofu mixture into a second saucepan and cook over medium heat for 10 minutes.

4. Now you're ready to put it all together. In a lightly greased lasagna pan, layer the ingredients. Start with a layer of noodles, then spinach, beans, tofu sauce, and tomato sauce. Repeat until all ingredients are used.

5. Top with Parmesan cheese and bake for 45 minutes, or until bubbly and golden brown on top.

6. Remove the lasagna from the oven, let stand for 5 minutes, and serve.

Makes 8 servings

Marinated Halibut

2–3 halibut fillets
1 cup Eggless Caesar Salad dressing (see Index)

1. Combine halibut and dressing in a small bowl, cover, and marinate in the refrigerator for 1 hour.
2. Preheat the oven to 350°F.
3. Place fish in a lightly oiled baking dish and bake for 11–15 minutes or until the fish is flaky.
4. Serve with Eggless Caesar Salad, Lemon Parsley Rice, and Asparagus with Red Pepper (see Index).

Makes 4 servings

Of Fats and Fish

The omega-3 fatty acids found in cold-water fish such as salmon, halibut, mackerel, whitefish, and lake trout reduce the risk of blood clots and may prevent the spread of cancer cells through the blood.

Salmon and Bok Choy over Rice

....

2 tablespoons miso dissolved in 2 cups water
1 cup brown rice
3 stalks bok choy, cut into ½-inch slices
1 pound fresh salmon

1. In a large saucepan, over medium-high heat, bring miso broth to a boil.
2. Add rice, lower heat, cover, and cook for 30 minutes.
3. Place bok choy on top of cooked rice, then place salmon on top of bok choy. Replace the lid and steam on low heat for 15 minutes, or until salmon is cooked through.
4. Serve with lemon wedges and Tofu Tartar Sauce (see Index).

~ Makes 2 servings

Salmon with Roasted Garlic and Rosemary

2 bulbs garlic, unpeeled
3 tablespoons fresh lemon juice
4 sprigs fresh rosemary *or* 1 teaspoon dried rosemary
¼ cup flaxseed oil
2 8- to 10-ounce fresh salmon fillets

1. Preheat the oven to 350°F.
2. Wrap the garlic bulbs loosely in aluminum foil and place directly on oven rack. Roast garlic for 45 minutes, or until the individual cloves are very tender. Test with a knife for doneness. Remove from the oven and let cool.
3. Peel the garlic, discarding the outer skin.
4. In a food processor combine garlic, lemon juice, rosemary, and oil. Puree until smooth.
5. Spread puree on top of salmon. Lightly oil a baking dish with canola oil. Place fish in the baking dish and bake until fish is flaky. This is also great cooked on the grill.

~ *Makes 4 servings*

A Healthy One-Two Punch

Salmon's essential fatty acids stimulate the immune system and inhibit tumor growth. Garlic protects the immune system and adds a rich complementary flavor to the salmon.

Salmon with Tofu

1 cup smooth tofu

6 cloves garlic, minced

1 teaspoon dill

Juice of 1 lemon

2 pounds salmon fillets

1 tablespoon extra-virgin olive oil

1. Preheat the oven to 350°F.
2. Place tofu, garlic, dill, and lemon juice in a food processor or blender and puree until smooth.
3. Pat the mixture evenly over the salmon.
4. Lightly oil a large baking dish with olive oil. Place the salmon in the baking dish and bake for 15 minutes, or until fish is flaky.

~ *Makes 4 servings*

Pasta with Clams

....

2 tablespoons extra-virgin olive oil

3 cloves minced garlic

½ teaspoon fennel seeds

½ teaspoon dried lemongrass

3 cups whole-grain pasta

2 6½-ounce cans clams with juice

1 8-ounce bottle clam juice

¼ cup sun-dried tomatoes

Juice of ½ lemon

2 tablespoons nutritional yeast

2 tablespoons chopped fresh parsley

1. Heat the olive oil in a sauté pan. Add the garlic, fennel seeds, and lemongrass and sauté over medium heat until lightly browned, about 20 minutes.
2. In the meantime, cook the pasta as directed on the package. Drain thoroughly and place in a large bowl.
3. Add the clams, clam juice, and tomatoes to the sauté pan and continue to cook gently until warmed through, about 3 minutes.
4. Pour the clam sauce into the bowl with the cooked pasta. Add the lemon juice, nutritional yeast, and parsley and toss gently. Serve immediately.

⌒ Makes 6 servings

Herbed Butter for Seafood

¼ cup extra-virgin olive oil
¼ cup softened butter
2 tablespoons chopped fresh dill
½ cup fresh lemon juice
½ teaspoon sea salt

1. Whisk the olive oil with the softened butter until the mixture is creamy.
2. Place the olive oil–butter mixture, chopped dill, lemon juice, and salt in a small saucepan. Cook over a low heat until the butter is melted.
3. Brush over fish or other seafood.

Makes about 1 cup

5

Soy Products

The soybean is one of the most versatile and nutritious foods you can eat. It is rich in protein, fiber, and minerals; low in saturated fat; and totally devoid of cholesterol. For centuries people have transformed this lowly bean into creamy tofu, liquid milk, firm tempeh, and salty condiments such as miso and tamari. Today soy products are also available in a multitude of flavored, preseasoned, and precooked forms. This wide variety of tastes and textures makes increasing the soy products in your diet a very easy and delicious task.

The nutritional benefits of soy products are the object of much research. Studies show that the following compounds, which are found in most soy products, can have a healthy impact on cancer treatment.

- Genistein, a phytoestrogen (estrogen-like compound produced in the intestines by bacterial action) that has antioxidant properties, may block the formation of new blood vessels in cancer tumors, and reduces the cancer-promoting effects of estrogen.
- Equol and daidzein are phytoestrogens that reduce the cancer-promoting effects of estrogen.
- Protease inhibitors are thought to prevent transformation of normal cells into malignancies.
- Saponins stimulate the immune system, inhibit specific types of cancer cells in vitro, and inhibit the replication of Epstein-Barr virus.

- Other antioxidants isolated from soybeans include caffeic acid, chlorogenic acid, and ferulic acid.

Populations that consume large amounts of soy foods, such as the Japanese and the Chinese, have significantly reduced incidence of specific types of cancer. Asian women who consume soy products regularly have lower rates of breast cancer than American women who do not consume soy. Colon cancer incidence is reduced by 50 percent in those whose diets include plenty of miso soup.

Miso

Miso is a fermented soybean paste, used to make the familiar salty soup served in Japanese restaurants. It is credited with many nutritional and health-promoting properties. Researchers have found that it decreases the risk of developing some forms of cancer and heart disease.

Miso has an incredible aroma not unlike fine wine and is available in a variety of flavors. Sweet miso (including mellow miso and white miso) is light in color and best used for delicate recipes such as dressings and cream soups. It can also serve as a dairy substitute in dips. Red miso (including rice miso, barley miso, and brown rice miso) is darker in color and saltier in taste than sweet miso; it is best used in hearty soups, stews, and gravies or as bouillon.

Soy Milk

Soy milk is made by a process that blends cooked soybeans with water and then strains off the solids. The result is a nutty-tasting protein-rich liquid. It is available in full-fat, reduced-fat, and flavored varieties and made by several different companies. Since it contains no lactose or milk protein, fortified soy milk can be used as a dairy milk substitute. Almost all companies sell soy milk in sterile packages that, when unopened, last for about a year in the cupboard. Once opened, soy milk is usually good for about a week.

Tamari and Shoyu

Tamari is natural soy sauce made from soybeans. Shoyu is a soy sauce made from equal amounts of soybeans and cracked wheat. These salty condiments are the basis for flavoring in many Asian dishes. They bring to recipes a distinctive Asian edge and rich flavor. Do not confuse these nutrient-rich natural products with common soy sauce, which is an artificial unfermented product.

Tofu

Tofu's growing popularity has created a market for a variety of products now widely available at most grocery stores. Tofu is a block of soybean curd. It has almost no flavor and will absorb any flavors added to it. It is highly nutritious, protein-dense, and rich in minerals and healthful fats.

Firm tofu is best for slicing, stir-frying, and simmering in soups and stews. Soft tofu has more water than the firm type and lends itself to creamy dips, dressings, and miso broth. Silken tofu is a custard-like product that is best used for desserts such as puddings, pies, and delicate sauces.

Tempeh

Tempeh (pronounced tem-*pay*) is made by inoculating split soybeans with a fungal culture. As the mold grows, it binds the soybeans together and partially breaks down the proteins, fats, and carbohydrates, making tempeh very easy to digest. Fresh tempeh has a wonderful mushroomy odor and a nutty flavor. It can be used as a substitute for beef, chicken, or pork in recipes.

Green Tea Miso Soup

4 cups strong brewed green tea
3 tablespoons finely chopped scallion
1 tablespoon nori-miso flakes
4 tablespoons miso

1. In a large saucepan, gently heat tea, scallion, and miso flakes until almost boiling.
2. Remove from heat and stir in miso. Serve immediately.

Makes 4 servings

Edamame-Steamed Soybean Pods

4 cups water
1 pound fresh or thawed soybean pods
1 teaspoon sea salt

1. In a large saucepan, bring water to a boil.
2. Secure a bamboo steamer over the top of the saucepan and place soybean pods in it. Steam for 15 minutes.
3. Sprinkle with sea salt and serve immediately.
4. To eat, pinch the pod and the beans will pop out, or pull the pod between your teeth to extract the beans.

Makes 4 servings

Soy Burgers

....

2 tablespoons extra-virgin olive oil

4 cloves garlic, sliced

2 medium yellow onions, minced

2 stalks celery, minced

½ medium green bell pepper, diced

½ cup diced carrot

1 teaspoon salt

½ teaspoon dried basil

½ teaspoon dried parsley

¼ teaspoon oregano

2 cups cooked soybeans

3 tablespoons miso dissolved in 1 cup water

2 cups cooked brown rice

2 tablespoons tahini (ground sesame seed paste)

2 tablespoons almond butter

1 egg, beaten

1 tablespoon canola oil

1. Heat the olive oil in a large pan. Add the garlic and onion and sauté over medium-low heat for 5 minutes.
2. Add the celery, bell pepper, and carrot. Stir in the seasonings and continue to sauté for an additional 5–10 minutes. Preheat the oven to 350°F.
3. While the vegetables are cooking, place the beans and miso broth in a blender or food processor. Process until beans are thoroughly mashed.
4. Add the beans and the rice to the vegetables and remove from heat.

5. In a small bowl, beat together the tahini, almond butter, and egg. Pour the egg mixture into the vegetables and mix together well.

6. Form the mixture into 8 patties. Lightly oil a cookie sheet with canola oil. Arrange the patties on the cookie sheet and bake for 20 minutes on each side. Loosen the edges carefully before turning over.

7. Serve on whole wheat hamburger buns with greens and Tofu Ketchup (see Index). Patties can be frozen for later use.

Makes 8 servings

Fresh Green Soybeans

1 pound fresh or thawed soybean pods
1 teaspoon sea salt

1. Place soybeans in a large bowl.
2. Bring one quart of water to a boil and pour it over the soybeans.
3. Let stand 5 minutes, then drain and cool. Break the pods and squeeze out the beans.
4. Using the same pan, boil 1 cup of fresh water. Add beans and salt and return to a boil.
5. Cover the pot and cook the beans at a low boil for 10-15 minutes. Drain and serve immediately.

~ *Makes 4 servings*

Tofu Scramble

....

1 teaspoon canola oil
1 teaspoon hot pepper oil (optional)
1 yellow onion, sliced
8 ounces firm tofu, crumbled
4 cloves garlic, sliced thin
½ cup broken dried seaweed, nori or dulse
1 teaspoon curry powder
½ cup nutritional yeast

1. Heat the canola and hot pepper oils in a skillet.
2. Add onion and tofu and sauté over medium heat until onion is translucent, about 5 minutes.
3. Reduce heat, add garlic, and stir gently until tofu is lightly browned, about 5 more minutes.
4. Stir in seaweed and curry powder and continue cooking until heated through.
5. Remove from heat, stir in nutritional yeast, and mash with a fork until mixture resembles scrambled eggs.
6. Serve immediately with whole-grain toast.

Makes 2 servings

Creamy Tofu Pasta

2 tablespoons extra-virgin olive oil
4 large cloves garlic, chopped fine
¼ cup finely chopped red onion
1 32-ounce package soft tofu
½ cup water
3½ tablespoons tamari
1½ teaspoons dried sweet basil
2 cups hot cooked pasta
¼ cup chopped fresh parsley

1. Heat the olive oil in a small pan. Add garlic and onion and sauté over medium-low heat until the onion is translucent.
2. In food processor, blend the tofu until it reaches a uniform consistency. Pour the blended tofu into sauté pan with the garlic and onion, and cook for 5 minutes over medium heat.
3. Add water, tamari, and basil to the pan and cook for 5 minutes more.
4. Pour the tofu sauce over cooked pasta. Toss well and sprinkle with parsley. Serve immediately.

Makes 4 servings

Mushroom Tofu Supreme

4 tablespoons sesame seeds

2 tablespoons extra-virgin olive oil

2 large yellow onions, sliced thin

8 cloves garlic, chopped fine

8 ounces firm tofu, cut into small cubes

1 pound mushrooms, sliced

1 teaspoon dried basil

1 cup chopped fresh parsley

2½ tablespoons miso

¾ cup water

1 cup frozen peas

2 tablespoons flaxseed oil (optional)

2 cups hot cooked pasta

1. In a small dry pan, toast the sesame seeds, stirring constantly until they begin to brown. Set aside.

2. Heat olive oil in a large pan. Add onion, garlic, tofu, and mushrooms and sauté over medium-low heat until onion is translucent.

3. Add basil, parsley, miso, and water and cook, stirring, for an additional 5 minutes.

4. Add frozen peas and cook until heated through.

5. Divide the cooked pasta into 4 serving bowls and top with vegetables.

6. Drizzle 2 teaspoons of flaxseed oil onto each serving, if desired. Sprinkle each serving with sesame seeds.

~ *Makes 4 servings*

Tofu Enchiladas

....

ENCHILADA SAUCE

1 tablespoon extra-virgin olive oil
1 medium yellow onion, minced
1 clove garlic, minced
1 28-ounce can stewed tomatoes
2 scallions, sliced thin
1 teaspoon red pepper flakes
1 teaspoon chili powder
1 teaspoon sea salt
½ teaspoon oregano
½ teaspoon cumin

ENCHILADAS

1 tablespoon extra-virgin olive oil
1 medium yellow onion, chopped fine
2 cloves garlic, minced
1 cup cooked black beans
1 10-ounce package silken tofu
10 corn tortillas
1 cup soy cheese, grated

To Make the Sauce

1. Heat the olive oil in a large saucepan. Add onion and garlic and sauté over medium-low heat until onion is translucent.
2. Add the remaining ingredients, cover, and cook over medium heat for 20 minutes.
3. Mash the tomatoes with a fork until the sauce is a fairly uniform consistency. Set aside while you make the enchiladas.

To Make the Enchiladas

1. Preheat the oven to 350°F.
2. Heat the olive oil in a large pan. Add onion and garlic and sauté over medium-low heat until onion is translucent, about 5 minutes.
3. Remove the pan from the heat and add beans and tofu to the onion mixture. Mash together with a potato masher. Set aside.
4. Dip each tortilla into the Enchilada Sauce, coating it completely. Roll each corn tortilla around ¼ cup of the bean mixture.
5. Lightly oil a large baking dish with canola oil. Arrange the rolled tortillas into the baking dish.
6. Pour the remaining enchilada sauce over the top and sprinkle with soy cheese.
7. Bake for 30 minutes.

Makes 10 enchiladas

Tofu Sauté

....

2 tablespoons canola oil

3 cloves garlic, crushed

1 tablespoon tamari

1 tablespoon minced ginger

1 tablespoon honey

1 16-ounce package tofu, sliced lengthwise

1 tablespoon sesame seeds

1. Heat the canola oil in a large skillet. Add the garlic and sauté over medium-low heat until translucent.
2. Add tamari, ginger, and honey and stir well.
3. Add slices of tofu, stirring to coat each slice and sauté until browned.
4. Add sesame seeds and serve hot with brown rice, or chill for a high-protein snack.

~ Makes 4 servings

Tofu "Meat" Balls

1 16-ounce package firm tofu, broken into pieces
2 eggs
½ cup bread crumbs
2 tablespoons bouillon *or* tamari
½ teaspoon onion salt
½ teaspoon Italian seasoning
½ teaspoon garlic powder
¼ cup freshly grated Parmesan cheese
1 tablespoon onion flakes
¼ teaspoon pepper
¼ teaspoon nutmeg
1 tablespoon extra-virgin olive oil *or* 1 tablespoon butter

1. Combine all ingredients except the oil or butter in a bowl. Mix well. Form into 1-inch balls.
2. Heat oil or butter in a large skillet. Add the tofu balls and sauté over medium-low heat until browned.
3. Serve with marinara sauce and pasta.

Makes 6 servings

Tempeh Herb Pasta

....

2 tablespoons sesame oil

3 tablespoons extra-virgin olive oil

1 tablespoon dried rosemary

1 teaspoon tarragon

¼ cup finely chopped yellow onion

2 cloves garlic, sliced

2½ cups water

3 tablespoons miso

¼ cup chopped fresh parsley

2 tablespoons finely chopped basil

½ pound tempeh, cut into ½-inch pieces (about 1 cup)

1 tablespoon tamari

2 cups hot cooked pasta of choice

½ cup Parmesan cheese

1. Heat the sesame oil and 2 tablespoons of the olive oil in a saucepan. Add rosemary, tarragon, onion, and garlic and sauté over medium heat until onion is translucent.

2. Add water and miso and simmer for 15 minutes. Add parsley and basil, stir, and set aside.

3. In a separate pan, heat the remaining tablespoon of olive oil. Add tempeh and tamari. Sauté over medium heat until the tempeh is browned.

4. Toss sauce and tempeh into pasta, sprinkle the top of each dish with grated Parmesan, and serve.

Makes 4 servings

Tofu Ketchup

4 ounces soft tofu

2 cups tomato sauce

1 tablespoon finely chopped yellow onion

1 teaspoon extra-virgin olive oil

1 teaspoon honey

1 teaspoon lemon juice

1. Place all ingredients in a blender or food processor.
2. Process on medium speed until creamy.

Makes 2 ½ cups

Tofu Tartar Sauce

4 ounces soft tofu
2 tablespoons lemon juice
1 tablespoon flaxseed oil
1 tablespoon chopped parsley
1 tablespoon fresh dill
¼ teaspoon hot mustard
Pinch of sea salt
½ cup finely chopped sweet pickle

1. Place all ingredients except the pickle in a blender or food processor. Process on medium speed until smooth.
2. Stir in the pickle. Refrigerate until ready to serve.

Makes about ¾ cup

Tofu Coconut Pudding

8 ounces silken tofu
1 tablespoon frozen orange juice concentrate
½ cup canned crushed unsweetened pineapple
½ cup grated unsweetened coconut
1 teaspoon coconut extract
¼ teaspoon freshly ground ginger

1. Combine all ingredients in a blender or food processor and process until smooth and creamy.
2. Serve chilled or unchilled in ½-cup servings.
3. Sprinkle additional grated coconut on top, if desired.

Makes 4 servings

6

....

Meals in a Glass

The "friendly fire" of cancer treatment often causes anorexia or loss of appetite. You know you should be eating more, but you just don't feel like it. At other times sores or rawness in the mouth and throat makes eating painful and swallowing difficult.

When you do not feel hungry or when eating provides more pain than pleasure, try one of the nutritious meal shakes in this chapter. Even when food is the farthest thing from your mind, a soothing drink can be welcome. Remember, even though you may not feel hungry, your cells still need nourishment to keep you healthy.

Where to Buy the Ingredients

All of the necessary ingredients for the recipes in this chapter can be purchased in health food stores or through distributors of nutritional products. In some parts of the country, supermarkets also have natural food sections that carry health foods.

A confusing array of protein powders and mixes is available. Be prepared to shop around, and always read the ingredient labels carefully. Protein powders intended for body builders and athletes often have serving sizes that contain very high levels of protein. These levels can stress your kidneys, so make sure to add only 10 to 15 grams of protein per shake,

unless your physician suggests otherwise. Some excellent protein powders are marketed as weight-loss drinks or meal-
replacement drinks. Many of these formulas are supplemented
with fiber.

You may want to purchase a brand that fulfills some of your
vitamin and mineral needs. This will decrease the number of
pills you have to swallow. Read the label and choose either a
whey protein source or a soy protein source. To avoid allergy
problems, do not buy protein drinks at the supermarket. They
may be dairy-based. Many people are allergic to dairy products or are lactose-intolerant. Store-bought formulas also often
contain large quantities of sugar and numerous protein
sources. When deciding on a protein supplement, take into
consideration any food allergies or intolerances.

Protein powders made from soybeans do *not* contain any of
the beneficial phytochemicals found in soy foods and are *not*
a substitute for soy foods. You may wish to add soy milk to
your drinks along with the protein powder. Eight ounces of
soy milk provides about 3 grams of protein.

The Basic Meal Shake

....

Breakfast shakes are a great way to begin the day when you are not used to eating breakfast, or for those mornings when you just don't feel like eating. This recipe offers carbohydrates to supply your immediate energy needs, protein to keep you awake and alert, healthy fats to aid in the absorption of fat-soluble vitamins and to build energy reserves, and fiber to keep your bowels functioning normally.

Liquid (1 cup) Juice, water, nonfat milk, nonfat yogurt, soy milk, rice milk, or nut milk.

Fruit (½ cup, chopped) Any soft fruit including bananas, strawberries, blackberries, blueberries, pineapple, and papaya. Frozen fruits make thicker shakes.

Flaxseed Oil (1–2 teaspoons) Fresh flaxseed oil is perishable. Look for it in the refrigerated food section and be sure to check the bottle's expiration date. Buy the brands that come in dark bottles. They are designed to protect the fatty acids from sunlight. Purchase the oil in small amounts and store in the refrigerator. Each teaspoon of oil adds 40 calories and 4½ grams of fat.

MCT Oil **(1–2 tablespoons)**	Medium chain triglyceride (MCT) oil is available without prescription from your pharmacy. The fats in MCT oil are easily digested and absorbed when other sources of fat are not. When you are trying to maintain weight or when you want to gain lost weight back, add this oil to shakes to increase your caloric intake. The taste of MCT oil is not very palatable, so start with a smaller amount of oil to accustom yourself to the taste. Each tablespoon of MCT oil adds 115 calories and 14 grams of fat.
Protein Powder **(10–15 grams)**	Preferably from a soy or whey protein powder.
Fiber Powder	An effective fiber blend will provide 5 grams of fiber from a *mixed* fiber source that is designed to dissolve in liquid. Since each type of fiber has unique benefits, choose a brand that contains at least three different sources of fiber. These products are often marketed as bulk laxatives, colon detoxifiers, and cholesterol reducers.

If you have difficulty swallowing pills, consider adding the following products to your shake.

Nutritional Yeast   Nutritional yeast is available as a powder that can be sprinkled on foods or mixed into drinks. It is a tasty source of chromium and all of the B vitamins and can replace a B-vitamin supplement.

Multivitamin   Use a powdered or liquid multivitamin-multimineral supplement *without iron* (supplementing iron can cause constipation for those who are not deficient). Put one half the day's recommended dosage in a shake.

Vitamin C   Adds extra vitamin C to drinks. Try an effervescent powder to put fizz and zest into your fruit drinks.

1. Add fruit, liquids, and oils to blender and process until smooth.
2. Sprinkle in the powdered ingredients and continue processing until thoroughly blended.
3. The ingredients tend to settle and separate, so it's best to drink the shake immediately.

∼ *Makes 1 serving*

Vanilla Breakfast Shake

The soy milk in this recipe is an excellent vegetarian source of phytochemicals (cancer-fighting, naturally occurring chemicals).

1 ripe banana, broken into pieces
6 ounces vanilla-flavored soy milk
1 teaspoon flaxseed oil
1 scoop vanilla-flavored protein drink powder (read the label to calculate the size the serving will need to be to include approximately 10 grams of protein)
1 tablespoon fiber mix (about 5 grams)
1 teaspoon high-chromium nutritional yeast

1. In a blender, layer fruit, then liquid ingredients, and then solid ingredients.
2. Process until smooth. Drink immediately.

Makes 1 serving

Chocolate Supreme Shake

....

It tastes too delicious to be nutritious, but this rich concoction is loaded with vitamins and minerals. For a higher-calorie drink, add more flaxseed oil or MCT oil.

½ cup fresh or frozen strawberries
6 ounces cocoa- or carob-flavored soy milk
1 teaspoon flaxseed oil
½ teaspoon high-quality unsweetened cocoa powder
1 scoop cocoa-, carob-, or chocolate-flavored protein
   powder (read the label to calculate the size the serving
   will need to be to include approximately 10 grams of
   protein)
1 tablespoon fiber mix (about 5 grams)

1. In a blender, layer fruit, then liquid ingredients, and
   then solid ingredients.
2. Process until smooth. Drink immediately.

Makes 1 serving

Pineapple and Cream Weight-Gain Shake

....

This is a recipe for those who wish to stop weight loss or to gain a few pounds. Add an additional tablespoon of MCT *oil for a higher-calorie drink.*

¾ cup cubed pineapple chunks
¾ cup coconut milk
1 tablespoon MCT oil
½ teaspoon pure vanilla extract
1 tablespoon fiber powder
1 scoop vanilla-flavored protein powder (read the label
to calculate the size the serving will need to be to
include approximately 10 grams of protein)

1. In a blender, layer fruit, then liquid ingredients, and
then solid ingredients.
2. Process until smooth. Drink immediately.

~ *Makes 1 serving*

Creamy Tomato Weight-Gain Shake

For those days when you don't feel like a sweet drink, here's a tasty alternative. For a higher-calorie drink, add more MCT oil or a tablespoon of flaxseed oil.

6 ounces low-sodium tomato juice
¼ cup nonfat plain yogurt
1 tablespoon MCT oil
1 scoop unflavored protein powder (10 grams protein)
1 tablespoon fiber powder
1 teaspoon nutritional yeast

1. Into a blender, place liquid ingredients and then solid ingredients.
2. Process until smooth. Drink immediately.

Makes 1 serving

Orange Cow

....

You can use this as an afternoon pick-me-up drink to complement the morning shake. If weight loss is not a problem, omit the MCT oil.

    1 cup nonfat yogurt
    2 tablespoons frozen orange juice concentrate
    1 tablespoon MCT oil
    10 grams unflavored protein powder
    ½ teaspoon powdered vitamin C
    1 tablespoon fiber mix (5 grams)

1. Into a blender, place liquid ingredients and then solid
   ingredients.
2. Process until smooth. Drink immediately.

⁓ Makes 1 serving

Blue Cow

....

This is a dairy-free version of the Orange Cow.

⅓ cup fresh or frozen blueberries
⅔ cup vanilla soy milk
1 tablespoon MCT oil
10 grams unflavored protein powder
1 tablespoon fiber mix (5 grams)

1. In a blender, layer fruit, then liquid ingredients, and then solid ingredients.
2. Process until smooth. Drink immediately.

~ *Makes 1 serving*

Chocolate Banana Smoothie

....

If your throat and mouth are sore, this makes a nutritious in-
between-meals snack. Garnish it with a thin slice of banana
notched over the rim of the glass.

  1 frozen banana, broken into pieces
  6 ounces fortified cocoa- or carob-flavored soy milk
  Large pinch of cinnamon

  1. In a blender, layer banana, soy milk, and then cinnamon.
  2. Process until smooth. Drink immediately.

∽ Makes 1 serving

Banana Nutmeg Smoothie

....

This is one of Maureen's favorite smoothie recipes. Dust the top with nutmeg just before serving.

   1 large ripe banana, broken into pieces
   6 ounces low-fat fortified vanilla soy milk
   ¼ teaspoon ground nutmeg

1. In a blender, layer banana, soy milk, and nutmeg.
2. Process until smooth. Drink immediately.

                                             Makes 1 serving

Berry Yogurt Smoothie

....

Cool and soothing, this shake is a good source of protein, calcium, and vitamin C. Use frozen strawberries that do not contain added sugar or syrup.

   6 ounces nonfat vanilla yogurt
   ½ cup frozen strawberries (or any frozen berry such as
      raspberries, blueberries, or a combination)
   ½ teaspoon pure vanilla extract

1. Place all ingredients in a blender and process until smooth.
2. Drink immediately.

~ *Makes 1 serving*

Sweet Almond Milk

....

Almond milk offers a nondairy alternative for drinking, mixing with protein powders for shakes, and pouring over cereals. You can also use it in baking and cooking. If you use it as a beverage, you'll want to strain it through cheesecloth first, as the milk is very pulpy.

- 1 cup almonds
- 3 cups cold water
- 1 tablespoon brown rice syrup
- 1 teaspoon pure vanilla extract

1. In a food processor fitted with a metal blade, grind almonds until very fine.
2. Place the ground almonds and the remaining ingredients in a blender and blend until creamy, white, and frothy.
3. Pour over hot or cold cereals or serve chilled.

⤳ Makes 4 servings

Almond Fruit Cup

....

*The almond milk can be made from the preceding Sweet Almond
Milk recipe or bought ready-made at your local health food store.
Rice milk also works well in this recipe.*

½ large ripe banana, broken into pieces
¼ cup frozen unsweetened strawberries
6 ounces Sweet Almond Milk
2 tablespoons frozen orange juice concentrate
1–2 drops pure almond extract

1. Add all ingredients to a blender.
2. Process until smooth.
3. Drink immediately.

Makes 1 serving

7

Juices

For centuries vegetable and fruit juices have been prized for their healing properties. The word *chemical* itself comes from the Greek word *chemia*, which means "plant juice." Fresh juices enable the cancer patient to enjoy the benefits of raw foods when chewing and swallowing are difficult and painful. When a low-fiber diet is all that can be tolerated, the only way a cancer patient can digest raw produce is in the form of juices.

To make juices you must have a fruit and vegetable juice extractor. A blender or appliance that pulverizes produce will not substitute.

Juicing Tips for Cancer Patients

- A little juice goes a long way. Two or three glasses a day is all you need to supplement your diet.
- Dark green leafy vegetables are strong tasting and should be diluted with other milder juices. Good mild juices on which to base a recipe include carrot, celery, cucumber, tomato, and cabbage.
- Be creative. Onions, leeks, garlic, horseradish, ginger, hot peppers, and fresh herbs can all be juiced.
- When the mouth and throat are painfully raw, avoid acidic juices such as tomato, pineapple, and citrus (orange, grapefruit, lemon, and lime).

- Never drink sweet juices on an empty stomach. This can raise blood sugar levels, and cancer cells love glucose. Sweet tastes can also cause nausea during chemotherapy and radiation therapy.
- Vegetable juices are best when consumed immediately. The juicing process mixes plant liquids with enzymes that start to break down the juice as soon as it reaches the glass.
- Citrus juices can be stored for up to 48 hours in a sealed container in the refrigerator. Juices made from melons (e.g., watermelon or cantaloupe) do not store well and should be consumed immediately.

Preparing Produce to Juice

- Buy organic produce when available.
- Wash all produce thoroughly with a nontoxic vegetable cleaner and rinse well.
- All nonorganic fruits and vegetables with a skin should be peeled.
- All nonorganic fruits and vegetables that are waxed (e.g., apples or cucumbers) should be peeled.
- Remove pits and stones before juicing. They can damage your machine.
- Remove apple and pear seeds before juicing. They contain small amounts of cyanide.

Power Orange Juice

Orange juice with an attitude! The white inner skin of the orange is rich in bioflavonoids. For a festive touch, use sparkling water.

2 oranges
Filtered water

1. Organic oranges can be juiced unpeeled. If your oranges are not organic, remove the orange's outer peel, leaving on as much of the white inner skin as possible.
2. Juice the oranges according to your machine's instructions. Add chilled filtered water to taste.
3. Drink immediately.

~ *Makes 1 serving*

Watermelon Breeze

....

Watermelon and tomatoes are the richest sources of lycopene, a carotenoid even more powerful than beta-carotene. If you do not like tomato juice or if your throat is too sore to drink acidic juices, this recipe provides an excellent way to get your lycopene. It helps to cool and soothe throats irritated by radiation or chemotherapy.

Watermelon slices (enough to extract 12 ounces of juice)

1. Peel skin, leaving only the green rind.
2. Juice the watermelon according to your machine's instructions. Don't worry about the seeds; they will be expelled with the pulp.
3. Pour juice into ice-filled glasses and drink immediately.

Makes 1 serving

Apple Juice Lite

This juice is good for tissues that have been injured by radiation and chemotherapy. Celery juice contains the same healing properties found in cabbage juice, while apple juice has antiviral properties. Apple juice is also a natural laxative.

2 apples, seeds removed
2 stalks celery, small leaves removed

1. Juice the apples and celery according to your machine's instructions.
2. Pour over crushed ice and drink immediately.

Makes 1 serving

Cantaloupe Combo

....

If you don't like carrots but still want the benefits of the carotenes, cantaloupe is a delicious alternative. This drink may remind you of a hot summer day when the lawn has just been mowed.

 1 large wedge of cantaloupe, rind removed
 2 stalks celery, small leaves removed

1. Juice the melon and celery according to your machine's instructions.
2. Drink immediately.

Makes 1 serving

Power Veggie Juice I

This is a powerhouse of cancer-fighting phytochemicals including carotenes, indoles, glucobrassicin, glutathione, and the isothiocyanates. Drink an 8-ounce glass each day. (See Chapter 12 in What to Eat if You Have Cancer.*)*

4 medium carrots
2 stalks celery, green leaves removed
4 large kale leaves

1. Juice the vegetables according to your juicing machine's instructions.
2. Drink immediately.

Makes 1 serving

Power Veggie Juice II

....

This is a special juice for those with hormone-dependent cancers such as prostate cancer, breast cancer, or ovarian cancer. Loose-leaf lettuce and bok choy are good sources of phytoestrogens (see Glossary), which help to detoxify estrogen in the liver, keeping circulatory levels low.

½ head loose-leaf lettuce
1 wedge bok choy (Chinese cabbage)
1 large broccoli spear
1 medium carrot

1. Juice the vegetables according to your juicing machine's instructions.
2. Drink immediately.

~ *Makes 1 serving*

The I-Can't-Believe-It's-Vegetable-Juice Juice

Here's a recipe for beginning juicers who hate vegetables. The sweetness of the carrots is balanced by the slightly salty taste of the celery. The lemon adds a surprising bright note that ties the flavors together.

4-6 medium carrots
2 stalks celery
1 small wedge lemon

1. Juice the vegetables and lemon according to your machine's instructions.
2. Drink immediately.

~ *Makes 1 serving*

Deluxe Tomato Juice

Tomatoes are one of the best sources of lycopene, a powerful antioxidant. The bell pepper enriches the flavor and adds even more vitamin C. If you find plain tomato juice bland and boring, try adding a thin slice of hot pepper to the juicer. The naturally occurring capsaicin in the pepper will wake up your mouth!

2 medium tomatoes
½ sweet red bell pepper

1. Juice the vegetables according to your juicing machine's instructions.
2. Drink immediately.

~ *Makes 1 serving*

Cucumber Cooler

Kale is an excellent source of calcium, magnesium, manganese, carotenoids, and vitamin C. This refreshing drink is an excellent choice when the mouth and throat are hot and irritated.

1 large cucumber, well chilled and then peeled
1–2 large kale leaves

1. Juice vegetables according to your juicing machine's instructions.
2. Pour into a chilled glass. Serve immediately.

Makes 1 serving

Beet Tonic

....

Beet root is traditionally considered a detoxifying juice. It is rich in potassium, folic acid, glutathione, and phytosterols.

    2 stalks celery, small leaves removed
    2 large kale leaves
    1 large beet, greens removed
    1 large carrot

1. Juice vegetables according to your juicing machine's instructions.
2. Pour into a chilled glass. Serve immediately.

Makes 1 serving

Tossed Salad

....

Don't feel like eating a salad? Drink *it instead. Romaine lettuce is an excellent source of calcium.*

½ medium head romaine lettuce
1 stalk celery
1 small tomato
1 medium carrot

1. Juice vegetables according to your juicing machine's instructions.
2. Pour into a chilled glass. Serve immediately.

⌒ Makes 1 serving

Coleslaw in a Cup

....

Cabbage is rich in the phytosterols that fight hormone-dependent cancers. Both cabbage and celery are known for their ability to speed the healing of sores in the stomach. This surprisingly mild juice is perfect for those being treated with chemotherapy and radiation.

¼ head cabbage
2 medium carrots
2 stalks celery, small leaves removed

1. Juice vegetables according to your juicing machine's instructions.
2. Pour into a chilled glass. Serve immediately.

~ *Makes 1 serving*

Recipes Using Juices

You can do more with juices than simply drink them. Use green juices made from low-oxalate vegetables (including kale, collard greens, turnip greens, cabbage, and dark green lettuces) to fortify other foods such as soups, stews, and sauces. When added to spicy, hearty dishes, they will not be noticed by the vegephobic. Kale juice is an excellent addition to tomato sauce. Celery juice perks up the flavor of soups. Add the juice just before serving so that the nutritive elements are not lost to heat.

Apple Ginger Tea

The ginger in this hot drink helps to reduce nausea associated with cancer treatment. Sip slowly. Grapefruit also works well as a substitute for the apple in this recipe.

½ apple with seeds removed
½-inch slice raw ginger
6 ounces very hot green tea

1. Juice the apple and ginger according to your machine's instructions.
2. Pour the juice into a mug and add hot tea.
3. Drink immediately.

~ *Makes 1 serving*

Instructions for Brewing Green Tea

Use 1 teaspoon tea leaves for a small pot of tea. Use 2 teaspoons tea leaves for a large pot of tea. Boil water, then pour into a porcelain teapot or mug and let cool for 1 minute. Add tea leaves. Let brew for 1 minute. Serve or add to juice immediately.

Evening Tonic

....

Apple juice is a natural laxative. Drink this juice just after your evening snack for relief of constipation. It tastes like warm apple pie.

   2 apples, seeds removed
   6 ounces boiling water
   Large pinch apple pie spice

1. Juice the apples according to your juicing machine's instructions.
2. Pour the juice into a large mug. Add boiling water and stir in the spice.
3. Drink immediately.

Makes 1 serving

Chilled Tomato Soup

....

This makes a light, nutritious meal, especially tasty for those with a small appetite. An onion slice can be substituted for the garlic clove. To add calories, brown the croutons in a tablespoon of extra-virgin olive oil.

1 large tomato
½ stalk celery
1 clove garlic
¼ cup nonfat plain yogurt
Salt and pepper to taste
½ cup seasoned whole-grain croutons

1. Juice the vegetables according to your juicing machine's instructions.
2. Pour into a bowl and dollop the yogurt in the center. Swirl yogurt with a knife.
3. Season to taste and garnish with a generous portion of croutons.
4. Serve immediately.

Makes 1 serving

Salad Splash

....

This is a wonderful seasoning for salads, steamed grains, or cooked vegetables.

   2 lemons
   1 medium onion

1. Juice lemons and onion according to your machine's instructions.
2. Use immediately or store in a clean covered jar in the refrigerator for up to two days.

Makes 2 servings

Juice Jelly

....

This is a soothing snack for someone with a sore throat or a light appetite.

    2 cups fresh fruit or berry juice
    1½ teaspoons granulated agar

1. Place juice in a small saucepan, sprinkle agar on top, and let sit for 2–3 minutes until agar is softened.
2. Over low heat, bring the juice to a simmer and stir until the agar dissolves, about 10 minutes.
3. Stir and cook for 5 additional minutes.
4. Pour into serving dishes and chill in refrigerator until thickened. Serve chilled.

Makes 2 servings

Juice Pops

....

One of the best medicines for throat and mouth irritation is ice.
Always keep a supply of these medicinal treats in the freezer.

  2 cups juice
  6 5-ounce paper cups or molds
  6 wooden ice-cream sticks

1. Divide the juice among the cups (fill a little less than
   ⅔ full) and place in freezer.
2. When ice starts to form, place a wooden stick in the
   center of each cup.
3. When juice pops have frozen solid, just remove the mold
   or cup.

                                          ~ *Makes 6 servings*

Things You Should Not Put into Your Juicer

- Apple and pear seeds (contain small amounts of cyanide)
- Carrot greens or tops (inedible)
- Celery leaves (taste very bitter)
- Stones or pits (will damage juicer)
- Bananas (contain no juice)
- Coconuts (cannot be juiced)
- Rhubarb (too high in oxalates)
- Frozen or thawed produce (cannot be juiced)
- Cooked produce (cannot be juiced)
- Nuts, seeds, or grains (will damage juicer)
- Beans (will damage juicer)
- Fingers (always push produce into juicer with the plunger provided by the manufacturer)

Mail-Order Companies

Arrowhead Mills
P.O. Box 2059
Hereford, TX 79045-2059

For a free product list, call (806) 364-0730 or fax (806) 364-8242. This quality company carries whole grains, nuts, seeds, beans, nut butters, oils, and mixes such as kamut pancake mix and blue corn waffle mix.

Bob's Red Mill–Natural Foods Inc.
5209 S.E. International Way
Milwaukee, OR 97222

For a free catalog, call (503) 654-3215 or fax (503) 653-1339. This company carries bean flours, barley products, whole grain hot cereals, corn products, dried fruits, flaxseed products, kasha, and rice products.

Deer Valley Farm
P.O. Box 173
Guilford, NY 13780-0173

For a free catalog, call (607) 764-8556. This company carries grains and seeds such as kamut, spelt, and quinoa.

Gold Mine Natural Food Company
3419 Hancock Street
San Diego, CA 92110-4307

For a free catalog, call (800) 475-3663 or fax (619) 296-9756. This company carries macrobiotic, organic, and Earthwise products. It features organic grains and beans. Gold Mine carries pressure cookers, miso, beans, soy sauce, sea salt, seeds, sea vegetables, seaweeds, whole grains, and oils.

Macrobiotic Company of America
799 Old Leicester Highway
Ashville, NC 28806

For a wholesale price list, call (800) 438-4730 or fax (704) 252-9479. Macrobiotic Company will send you details about all the high-quality products it carries, among them sea vegetables, gamasio, pressure cookers, sea salt, organic rice, tamari, shoyu, dried shiitake mushrooms, miso, and tofu.

Mountain Ark Trading Company
P.O. Box 3170
Fayetteville, AR 72702

For a free catalog, call (800) 643-8909 Monday through Friday 8:30 A.M. to 5:30 P.M. (Central Time) or fax (501) 521-9100. This company specializes in natural, organic, and macrobiotic foods. It carries such products as tempeh, tofu, barley malt syrup, black soybeans, and sesame oils.

Uwajimaya
519 6th Ave. South
Seattle, WA 98104

For a free catalog, call (800) 889-1928. This Asian market carries an extensive array of macrobiotic products and kitchen tools. It is very helpful in locating and mailing special items.

Walnut Acres Organic Farms
Walnut Acres Road
Penns Creek, PA 17862

For a free catalog, call (800) 433-3998. Walnut Acres Organic Farms offers a complete line of natural products and kitchen tools, including unrefined sugars, juicers, organic fruits and vegetables, canned soups, cookies, and rice cookers.

Glossary

Amaranth: This tiny seed is creamy beige in color and has an earthy flavor. It can be cooked as a hot cereal or ground into a flour and used in baked goods. Add to any grain, soup, or stew recipe.

Arugula: See **Rocket**.

Barley malt sweetener: The rich flavor of barley malt syrup complements baked goods and gives a protein shake an old-fashioned malt flavor. Barley malt is made from sprouted whole barley and can be purchased as a thick syrup or a dried powder.

Brassica: This is another name for vegetables in the cruciferous family.

Brown rice syrup: This sweetener is made from whole grain brown rice and sprouted barley. It has a delicate flavor and is especially good in hot tea and baked goods.

Buckwheat (kasha): A pale three-cornered seed, buckwheat is not related to wheat and is technically not even a grain. Mild in flavor and very quick cooking, it can be substituted for any grain. When roasted, it acquires its characteristic earthy flavor and is referred to as *kasha*. Buckwheat contains the flavonoid rutin, which is a powerful antioxidant.

Bulgur wheat (ALA or bulghur): Bulgur is cracked wheat berries that have been lightly cooked and parched (dried or roasted) and cracked. It cooks very quickly.

Carob: A popular chocolate alternative, this powdered tropical pod is rich in natural sugars, protein, calcium, and minerals.

Couscous: This is a type of pasta made from high-protein, whole durum wheat kernels that have been ground into flour. It is very quick cooking and comes out fluffy, light, and mild in flavor. Buy only whole wheat couscous.

Crucifers: A group of vegetables from the cabbage family, crucifers include cabbage, broccoli, and cauliflower.

Fortified soy milk: Soy milk is now fortified with vitamins just as dairy milk has been for years. Small amounts of the inexpensive fat-soluble vitamins A, D, E, and K are added as an extra measure, mainly for children who may be at risk for deficiency of these vitamins because of vegetarianism or malnutrition.

Gamasio: A traditional Japanese seasoning, gamasio is made by crushing together toasted sesame seeds and salt. It is a condiment that can be sprinkled on grain and bean dishes, soups, and salads.

Garbanzo beans (chickpeas): Rich in iron and a good source of unsaturated fats and fiber, these beans can be purchased in packages or in the bulk foods department of most grocery stores.

Jicama: A fleshy underground tuber (pronounced *hee*-ka-ma), this versatile vegetable has a crunchy texture somewhat like that of water chestnuts. Asian and Latin American markets as well as many grocery stores carry fresh jicama in the produce department. It has a light, sweet flavor, is ivory in color, and is juicy when fresh. The only preparation needed is the peeling of the tan skin. The flesh can be eaten raw or cooked.

Lentils: The lentil is a small legume that cooks quickly and does not require presoaking. Lentils come in several colors but all are nutritionally equal.

Millet: A small, beadlike grain with a slightly nutty flavor, millet is a good source of protein, thiamin, riboflavin, niacin, pyridoxine, and folate. The minerals magnesium, zinc, copper, and iron are also abundant in this native of Africa and Asia.

Mirin: This is a sweet Japanese rice cooking wine. It is often used to flavor white rice for making sushi.

Miso: A fermented soybean paste, miso is made by combining cooked soybeans with a fungus culture (koji), salt, and various grains, and letting the mixture ferment for from 6 months to several years. There are a number of major types available:

- Barley miso (*mugi*), which comes in two basic varieties, regular and sweet barley miso.
- Chinese *chiang*, the Chinese equivalent of Japanese miso made with wheat (*tien-m'ien chiang*) or red pepper (*la-chiao chiang*).
- Red miso, which is mild in flavor.
- Brown miso, which is fermented longer than red miso and is stronger in flavor.
- Rice miso (*kome*), which is made from soybeans and rice. It is sweet and delicate in flavor. Its basic varieties include red, light-yellow, semisweet beige, sweet red, and sweet white miso.
- Vegetable miso, which is relatively sweet in flavor and comes in several varieties—*kinzanji* miso, *moronomi* miso, *hishio*, and *namemiso*.

Nutritional yeast: This is a type of dried killed yeast. It can be purchased in most health food stores. It is rich in B vitamins and protein. Sprinkle it on top of dishes as you would Parmesan cheese.

Phytochemicals: Bioactive chemicals that are found in plants. See Chapter 12, "Phytochemicals and Cancer," in *What to Eat if You Have Cancer* for more information.

Phytoestrogens: Estrogen-like compounds present in plants. They reduce the risk of breast cancer.

Quinoa: Originally from the South American Andes, quinoa (pronounced *keen*-wah) is one of the best sources of protein in the plant kingdom. It is a delicious and quick-cooking grain with a mild flavor and a light beige color. Quinoa also contains substantial amounts of riboflavin, alphatocopherol, and carotenes.

Rocket (arugula): This is a mustard-flavored leafy green vegetable. Its bitter flavor encourages the release of digestive enzymes, thereby aiding in the digestive process. It also contains beta-carotene, vitamin C, calcium, and fiber.

Sea salt: This mineral-rich salt is sun-dried or kiln-baked. It has more flavor than regular table salt.

Sea vegetables/seaweed: These are marine plants rich in minerals such as calcium, iodine, and iron; vitamins; and amino acids. They are usually sold in dehydrated strips that can be broken or cut with scissors and softened by soaking for 20–30 minutes in warm water. Cook them along with beans, grains, and vegetables or cook them separately for 1–2 hours covered with water or until soft. They can also be roasted then ground into a fine powder with a coffee grinder for use as a condiment. Types of sea vegetable include:

- Arame, a dark yellow-brown sea vegetable rich in iron and calcium.
- Dulce, a purple-leaf sea vegetable that contains concentrated amounts of iodine, iron, and manganese.
- Hijiki, a stringy black sea vegetable rich in calcium, iron, iodine, riboflavin, and niacin.
- Kelp, a dried seaweed sold as a finely ground powder. It has a delicate salty flavor and is a good source of potassium, iodine, calcium, phosphorus, iron, and magnesium.
- Wakame, an olive-colored salty sea vegetable that grows in winglike fronds. It is a rich source of calcium, niacin, thiamin, and trace minerals.
- Nori, a tender seaweed commonly used for rolling sushi. It is the most easily digested of the seaweeds and is rich in beta-carotene, thiamin, and niacin.

Shiitake: This is a type of dried mushroom imported from Japan for its ever-increasing U.S. market. The shiitake is rich and earthy in flavor. There has been tremendous media attention focused on recent medical studies of the shiitake's anti-cancer properties.

Shoyu: Similar to soy sauce and tamari, this dark liquid is made from fermented soybeans and wheat.

Soy sauce: This is a black salty sauce made from wheat and soybeans.

Sucanat®: This is a trade name for a dehydrated organically grown sugarcane product. It is much less refined than white table sugar and contains some of the sugar cane's natural minerals and vitamins.

Tahini: This is a smooth paste made of ground sesame seeds.

Tofu: This is a soybean curd. It can be purchased in many different varieties—high fiber, reduced fiber, and reduced fat in soft, firm, or silken textures. It is an excellent source of protein and calcium.

Teff: This is a tiny dark brown grain with a light, nutty flavor. Roast it in a dry pan and add it to rice recipes.

Index